Weight Loss Surgery

FINDING THE THIN PERSON HIDING INSIDE YOU!

By Barbara Thompson

Third Edition

Disclaimer

This book was written and published strictly for informational purposes, and in no way should it be used as a substitute for consultation with your medical doctor, surgeon or health care professional. The facts in this book are based upon the author's experience and research and do not imply that your experience will be the same. The author is providing you the information so that you will be better able to choose, at your own risk, whether to act upon that information. You should not consider educational material herein to be the practice of medicine or to replace consultation with a physician or other medical practitioner.

All brand or product names mentioned in this book are the trademarks of their respective holders.

Word Association Publishers
205 Fifth Avenue
Tarentum, Pennsylvania 15084
800-827-7903
www.wordassociation.com

Cover designed by Roberta Colombari

ISBN 1-932205-30-6
Library of Congress Control Number: 2003101133

Table of Contents

Acknowledgements

Weight loss surgery is not a journey that you take alone. Many people along the way have been there for me, and this is my opportunity to let them know how much this has meant to me.

First of all, I would like to acknowledge Dr. Jorge Vazquez of Allegheny General Hospital in Pittsburgh, PA. Dr. Vazquez was the first doctor that I encountered who did not make me feel that my morbid obesity was my fault. He was the first doctor I knew who truly saw morbid obesity for the horrible, debilitating disease that it is, and was the first to have the courage and foresight to recommend weight loss surgery to me.

And I would like to thank Dr. Philip Schauer, of the University of Pittsburgh Medical Center. Dr. Schauer is a truly skilled surgeon, a leader in the field of bariatric surgery, and a compassionate human being who gave me my life back. He rejoices daily in the success of his patients and dedicates himself to their welfare. I am truly honored that he has consented to write the foreword to this book.

I would also like to thank my psychologist, Dr. Paul Friday, from Shadyside Hospital in Pittsburgh, PA. Dr. Friday hypnotized me for my surgery, was present during my surgery and my hospital stay, and helped my healing through his therapeutic messages.

As I went down the path on my journey to a new life, I was extremely fortunate to meet Linnann and Terry, who were both seeking a new life as well. From that point, the three of us continued together. We held hands across the Internet, encouraged each other, offered advice, laughed, moaned, and rejoiced for each other. I want to thank you both for your friendship and support.

In preparing this book, I received wonderful help and support. My very good friend, Joyceann Ditka took her time to proofread the manuscript as did my sister, Kathleen Moschetta. My sister also gave me encouragement and support during my whole weight loss experience. Dr. Schauer's bariatric nurse, Ms Beth Klemm, and his physician's assistant, Bill Gourash, edited the content of the manuscript. I would like to thank Jodie Auliff, OTR/L, Rehabilitation Institute of Chicago, for her contribution regarding occupational therapy. And to Tom Costello of Word Association, I give you my thanks for your enthusiasm over this project and helpful suggestions.

I want to thank my daughter, Erin, who patiently understood that I was ill and that my sometimes shortness with her came from pain, and not from my not loving her. She is so wise for such a young person.

And a very special thanks goes to my wonderful husband, life-partner and best friend, Frank, who supported my decision, stayed by my side in the hospital, cared for me at home, and loves me no matter what I look like. Frank has been invaluable in this project. He has edited this manuscript, encouraged this book, made wonderfully creative suggestions and picked up the slack for me when I was waist high in research material. Frank, I thank God for having you in my life.

And thank you to all of those online friends who have shared their experiences and advice. I have learned so much from each and every one of you. I have learned from your success and your struggles. You are anonymous friends, but friends nonetheless.

And I want to thank my Guardian Angel who has always helped me to discover the positive message in any adversity that I have ever experienced.

To all of you who take this weight loss journey, I applaud your courage and wish you safe harbor.

Should you want to contact me, reach me through my website at http://www.wlscenter.com or email me at barbara@wlscenter.com

Foreword

Bariatric surgeons often refer to weight loss surgery as a very powerful "tool" to help patients win the battle against severe obesity. In our bariatric surgery center at the University of Pittsburgh we, as do many bariatric surgeons, provide an "owner's manual" for patients to serve as a comprehensive instruction guide for their new tool. Just like the manufacture's instruction guide to a new computer program or an electronic device, the doctor's "instruction guide" although very informative, can sometimes be difficult to understand with some important information left out. For this reason, local bookstores are full of hot selling, practical instruction guides written by users who really know how the device works as opposed to the manufacturer. Well, Barbara Thompson's book just may be the first practical "owner's manual" for bariatric surgery written for and by the user (patient).

Barbara, who herself had laparoscopic gastric bypass surgery by myself and my partner, Dr. Sayeed Ikramuddin, begins by guiding the reader through that big step in deciding to have surgery and then how to choose a surgeon. She then discusses, in a very straightforward manner, the various operations available along with comparative advantages and disadvantages. This is followed by a very realistic description of what to expect during the hospital stay and during recovery. Some excellent advice is provided to help make the journey as safe and smooth as possible. The section on adjusting to new, healthy eating habits after surgery is full of very useful and practical guides that we often teach as well in our surgical weight loss clinic and support group meetings. She continues with some very practical suggestions on how to cope with and maintain success. We surgeons often forget that coping with success can be a challenge, and Barbara aptly addresses that issue. The final chapter written by her husband, Frank, is a must read for patient's family members and "significant others" for it poignantly addresses some of the anxieties and concerns held by loved ones who may have strong doubts about weight loss surgery based on ignorance.

Although Barbara clearly indicates that she is speaking as a layperson and not a medical professional, I found the medical information quite accurate and balanced with many references to reputable medical literature. She has appropriately indicated that expert opinion differs on some surgical issues such as choice of operation and the relative benefit of laparoscopic vs. open surgery. This book will indeed arm patients with very important information allowing them to be an active participant with their surgeon in making important decisions regarding their choice of operation. I am sure the reader will find Barbara's personal journey through weight loss surgery very real, genuine, and refreshing recognizing that individual experiences, as Barbara points out, may vary.

Ms. Thompson's book, <u>Weight Loss Surgery: Finding the Thin Person Hiding Inside You</u>, fills a critical void for patients who have had or are thinking about having weight loss surgery. She condenses an enormous volume of information from a larger variety of reputable sources into a very readable and understandable text. Her book provides a very practical guide to weight loss surgery written by a woman who not only knows how to use her tool effectively but also knows how to communicate effectively to people like herself who have struggled with severe obesity. In summary, it is a superb, comprehensive guide to weight loss surgery that I will recommend to all my patients and their primary physicians. Her success in winning the battle against obesity and writing this enormously valuable book is my reflected glory.

January 27, 2001
Phil Schauer, MD
Director of Bariatric Surgery
Director of Endoscopic Surgery
Department of Surgery
University of Pittsburgh
Pittsburgh, PA
412-647-2800

Introduction

After I found out from my doctor that I might need weight loss surgery, I was determined to find out all I could on this subject so that I could make the best decisions for me and become totally informed about this life-changing procedure. It has been a tremendous learning experience that continues to this day. Being a librarian, college faculty member, and a professional researcher, I had all of the resources available to me to do this research. I found out very quickly that the information is out there, but nowhere is it brought together in one place. So I decided to write this book. I hope it helps you as you go through your own journey to a healthier, thinner life. This book will answer basic questions that are asked time and time again and will provide you with non-medical advice that will allow you to talk to your surgeon with confidence and knowledge and help you decide if weight loss surgery is for you. It is not by any means meant to replace your doctor. I am very sure that this book will provide you with the information you will need to consult with your doctor regarding your own situation. I cannot stress enough how important it is to seek medical advice when you have medical questions.

Always, always discuss medical questions with medical personnel.

This book is written from a woman's point of view (because that's what I am) and it deals with some issues that are only applicable to women, such as an inability to get pregnant and what do I do about acrylic nails during surgery. However, most of this book is equally applicable to men as well. Many men have this surgery, and I don't want you men to believe that you are being ignored. Although most of this book is directed toward the Roux en-Y (RNY) surgery, much of the material is also applicable to Vertical Banded Gastroplasty (VBG) surgery or Duodenal Switch surgery, all of which I will describe in detail. I suggest that you use this book as a guide to prepare yourself to have the surgery and for living your life afterwards. I sincerely hope that by reading this book, you will be more successful with the entire weight loss surgery process by not making mistakes along the way.

Please remember that I am not a physician, nor am I a medical professional. I am a layperson who has first-hand knowledge of the procedure and did a tremendous amount of research to prepare myself for it. I have also continued to be involved in the weight loss surgery online arena. I continue to contribute and stay aware of what people having this surgery are questioning. If you do opt for the surgery, be sure that you communicate with your physician and use this book as a guide to ask questions. Your knowledge about the weight loss surgery procedure and how it will affect the rest of your life will make fear of the unknown disappear for you.

I know, from my own experience, what it is to go through all of the physical and emotional trials and joys of this surgery. Dr. Philip Schauer, from Pittsburgh, Pennsylvania, performed my surgery. I was blessed to have such a skilled and compassionate surgeon who gave me my life back. Although I had a few problems, I would do this again in a heartbeat. It is the best thing that I ever did for myself. Weight loss surgery is not for everyone, but it was my answer, and it may be yours as well.

1
My Important Decision

After years of steadily gaining weight, in October of 1998, my primary care physician referred me to a nutritional physician, Jorge Vazquez, M.D., who is the Director of Nutrition at Allegheny General Hospital in Pittsburgh, Pennsylvania. After reviewing my past history of many years of unsuccessful dieting and regaining weight, and my current physical condition, Dr. Vazquez was prepared to outline several courses of treatment for me. Before doing this, however, he needed to know how much weight I wanted to lose.

No doctor had ever asked me that before. Every doctor that I have ever been to had always said that I needed to lose weight, and the way to do it was to eat less and to exercise more (as if I didn't already know that!). But Dr. Vazquez asked me to decide what my goal was. Did I want to lose 5 percent of my weight, 10 percent, 20 percent, or 45 percent? Five percent would mean that at my weight of 264 pounds, I would then weigh 251 pounds. That was not acceptable to me. I might as well still weigh 264 pounds. With a 10 percent weight loss, I would weigh 238 pounds. That still wasn't close to where I wanted to head. I admitted to him that I wanted to lose it all. I wanted to be slim. "That was where I wanted to aim," I said confidently. It felt wonderful to admit that, to say it out loud. I wanted to be slim.

"Fine," said Dr. Vazquez, and he then proceeded to outline the treatment that would get me there. He explained that if I wanted to lose 5 percent of my weight, he would recommend diet and exercise. If I wanted to lose 10 percent of my weight, he would prescribe medications such as Meridia or Xenical. And if I wanted to lose 45 percent of my weight, I would have to have weight loss surgery! Whatever course of treatment I chose was fine with him. Dr Vazquez presented the three weight loss strategies in a very calculated and logical manner. It was totally up to me to select the course of action based on what I wanted as an outcome.

I suddenly understood that all of my adult life, I had been trying to beat the odds. I was trying to become slim and stay that way using methods that I had no statistical chance of achieving. Diet and exercise alone would never work. And I was living proof of that. The best that I could attain using the traditional method of diet and exercise was a 5 percent weight loss.

I felt like I was a contestant on Let's Make A Deal. Behind Door # 1 (diet and exercise) was Barbara weighing 251 pounds, looking about the same. Behind Door #2 (medication) was Barbara weighing 237 pounds, wearing a size 22 instead of a size 24. And behind Door #3 (weight loss surgery) was Barbara weighing 145 pounds wearing a size 10, slinky evening gown. I wanted to choose Door #3, but I didn't know if I was prepared to take on the risk of weight loss surgery?

I was in denial. How could I have let myself get to the point where my weight was so out of control?

Surgery! Wow! Did I dare open that door? And I questioned first how weight loss surgery was even an option for me. Wasn't weight loss surgery only performed on those who were over 400 pounds? Did I really qualify for weight loss surgery? I was shocked to find out that I was medically categorized as "morbidly obese." Yes, I knew I was overweight, OK maybe even fat. But I was now not only considered obese, but at 5'6" tall weighing 264 pounds, I was morbidly obese! How did I ever get this way? I was an expert on dieting and nutrition. How was it that I could be such a failure and be so weak that I could let myself become morbidly obese? While I was successful in every other aspect of my life, how could I let my weight get so out of control? How could I be such a failure at something I had worked so hard at for so many years? As I left Dr. Vazquez's office, my head was reeling.

I never thought that weight loss surgery would apply to me. I never even considered it. But the scale wasn't lying. My shock was so overwhelming that I wasn't yet ready to accept surgery as a solution. But the more I thought about it, the more intrigued I became. I knew that yet another diet would not work for me. Diets never had in the past. And now a doctor was telling me that the only way to successfully deal with my weight was through surgery. On my way home from the doctor's office, I stopped at the mall and walked past Victoria's Secret. I looked in the window and imagined myself wearing that beautiful lingerie. I actually felt lighter. Could being thin really be possible for me? Not just losing a few pounds that I would immediately regain, but I could lose it all and actually be slim forever! This was too much to imagine. Could Dr. Vazquez's Door #3 be a reality?

When I arrived home, I talked it over with my husband, explaining what Dr Vazquez had told me about my weight and the possibility of surgery. My husband was absolutely terrified about my having a surgical procedure that was so serious. He asked me to please just try one more diet, promising to help me and encourage me anyway he could. I could not blame him. We had been married less than four years at that time, so he had not experienced the years of diet failure that I had been through. So I conceded, and agreed to try one more diet. I went to a behavior modification and nutrition class every Monday night for four months. Along with the classes, I was prescribed the medication Meridia, and with this combination, I managed to lose 40 pounds. But six months after the class, the weight started to come back. All through this time, I was suffering with intense lower back pain. I took six to eight ibuprophen per day and went to a chiropractor several times a week. I also went to a pain clinic where I had three treatments of injections. Although the shots did provide me with some temporary relief, the doctor made it very clear that my back would not significantly improve unless I lost my excess weight. Throughout this time, I was studying weight loss surgery by reading everything I could get my hands on and talking to people who had the procedure themselves.

By the early Fall of 1999, I had regained the 40 pounds I had lost through my behavior modification class and prescribed medication, plus ten additional pounds and I was living with chronic back pain. I had reached a point at which I was having trouble working because my back would not hold out for a full day. Grocery shopping was agony and I could not take my twelve-year old daughter shopping for clothes. The pain was so intense that it affected my personality. It got to the point that when I would snap at my daughter, she would look at me and say, "Your back is really bad, isn't it, Mom?" She was so understanding. One night, with tears in my eyes, I said to my husband that I couldn't continue living with all this pain and had to go forward with the surgery. He understood and has become my biggest supporter through this whole process. My journey was just beginning!!

2
The Days of My Surgical Journey

I Can't Wait For The Big Day...

I am asked so often what I went through prior to my surgery. How did I feel and was I nervous? This is something that I must admit that I hate to talk about. I would like to say that I was completely calm about the coming surgery. I would like to say that through my research and careful consideration that I knew for sure that this was the path for me. I wish I could tell you that I headed into the surgery with confidence. Unfortunately, that did not describe me because I was a total wreck. I never had any type of surgery before and had only been in a hospital for a very short stay for bronchitis. My daughter is adopted, so I had not even gone through childbirth. I didn't have any prior experience with surgery so I had no idea what to expect. I was afraid of the pain. Heck, I was afraid that I might die! What would my life be like after this? What would it feel like to eat? Could I really give up the food that was my lifelong friend and great comfort? But as frightened as I was, I couldn't have the surgery come fast enough. I was impatient almost to the point of being breathless. I was totally hysterical.

I was afraid. I was hysterical. And I was eating everything in sight.

And through it all, I ate and ate and then ate some more! I went on a three month eating binge as I awaited my surgery. I had the last supper syndrome in a very big way. I was afraid that I would never be able to eat blackberry pie again, so I ate lots of blackberry pie. And how about quesadillas? I remember one evening, when I was having dinner with my husband. I started weeping over my wonderful que-sadilla, fearing that it was the last I would ever eat. I ate big greasy hamburgers. I ate french fries in my car everywhere that I went. I went through a virtual United Nations buffet. I ate Greek food, Chinese food, Italian food, Mexican food, Polish food, and French food. If it was food, I wanted to make sure I had it because in my mind, I was afraid it would be the last I would ever have. Consequently I gained over 20 pounds in 3 months. When the time finally came for my actual "last meal" before my surgery, I was so sick of food that I couldn't even eat it.

And how would I deal with eating after my surgery? I loved to eat. I loved the taste of food. I loved going out to dinner and enjoying all the great neighborhood restaurants as well as those when we would travel. I loved to cook and I loved using food in a nurturing way. Was I willing to give all that up? I thought about it. I pondered it. I feared it. Losing my good friend, food, was constantly on my mind. Food had been a central part of my life and I knew that through surgery, this would change. Was I willing to accept that change? I knew that as much as I loved food, it was destroying me. My friend of a lifetime was slowly but surely betraying me and I knew that I had to get it under control or I could never be happy.

Because my surgery was scheduled for late January, one of my fears was catching a cold or the flu. I was fearful that I might end up too sick to have my surgery if I did. Winter ailments run rampant in Pittsburgh, so I knew that I was especially susceptible, even though I had gotten my annual flu shot. I avoided crowds, washed my hands often, and took vitamin C and Echinacea. But on January 2nd, I came down with a terrible cold. I then proceeded to cough for the next three weeks. The day of my pre-surgery check-up, I sucked on a steady supply of cough drops, hoping that my surgeon's staff would-n't notice my constant hacking. Fortunately my lungs were clear and I didn't have a terrible cold after all. The cough was coming from a sinus infection. I was cleared for surgery even though I had the cough. But I still worried how I would manage to recover from surgery while I was coughing so badly. It sounded awfully painful to me!

Since I was having a major, intestinal surgical procedure done, I was required to do several preparatory tasks at home before arriving for my surgery. Some surgeons require more tasks than others, depending on what surgical procedure will be done, so you will need to ask for complete and accurate details from your surgeon of what you should do. What I am describing here is what I went through for my own RNY operation.

My preparation involved drinking clear liquids beginning two days prior to surgery. This included drinking only ginger ale, clear broth, Jello and juices, which seemed to satisfy me. I was very concerned about having only clear liquids and nothing else for those two days. I was sure that I would have cramps from being so hungry or would have headaches. I was dreading this fasting because I was afraid that I would be ravenously hungry. Since I always believed that real hunger was the most severe pain that anyone could endure, I have always had a fear of being hungry. I think it was all those stories about the poor starving people in _____ (You fill in the blank. It could be China, Africa, or whatever country your parents told you about to get you to clean your plate). As it turned out, I was fine. I had consumed so many "last suppers" that I was actually sick of food. Of course, from midnight prior to my surgery, I was not permitted anything by mouth.

> *I feared fasting before surgery so much.*
> *That is how strong my food addiction was.*

On the first day of the two days of preparation, I drank a bottle of Fleet Phospho Soda in order to have a bowel cleansing. I had to drink half of this, along with a glass of water, twice during that day, three hours apart. If you have ever done this in the past, you will know that it is not that bad. Fleet Phospho Soda has a slight citrus taste and is certainly potable. And the soda is very effective. That is a day when you definitely want to stay close to the bathroom throughout the day. Others have reported that they have had to use a product called

GoLitely. This has the same effect; it is just a larger quantity to drink. That day was not as bad as I expected and I thought that I was home free. Not so!

On the second day of my preparation, I was required to take a series of three antibiotics. I thought this would be easy but as it turned out, it was far worse than drinking the Fleet Phospho Soda. They were terrible. The antibiotics worked in my intestinal tract to kill any bacteria present, and were very hard on my stomach. They burned and made me so sick. I took one at 4:00 PM, one at 7:00 PM and one at 10:00 PM. By 9:00 PM, I was so sick that all I wanted to do was go to sleep, but couldn't because I had that last pill to take at 10:00 PM. It was not a pleasant day, but it did take my mind off my upcoming surgery.

That night, I also had to bathe using an antibacterial soap such as Dial, Lever 2000 or Hibiclens. When I got up the morning of my surgery, I had to bathe again using the antibacterial soap. I was then ready to leave for the hospital. I was anxious and nervous at the same time.

By the way, as if by magic, my cough disappeared that very morning

The Big Day...

I arrived at the hospital bright and early on the morning of Tuesday January 25th, 2000. My surgery was scheduled for 7:30 AM, so of course I was directed to arrive two hours earlier. The January weather in Pittsburgh, Pennsylvania, can be very tricky. We have had winters with just a little snow and other winters when the snow just would not stop. I had no idea what January 25th, 2000 would bring, but I knew that I didn't want anything to keep me from having this surgery. As an extra precaution, I reserved a room at a hotel near the hospital. If a heavy snowfall was predicted, my husband and I could arrive at the hotel the day before my surgery and then walk to the hospital in the morning. I of course assumed that, in the event of a snow storm, my surgeon would be able to make it, as well as all his surgical staff! I listened closely to the weather forecast the day before surgery and was relieved to learn that there was not a flake in sight. I was happy to cancel my hotel reservation.

After arriving at the hospital, I checked in and was assigned to a holding cubicle. Here I was weighed and my vital signs were checked. I was then given a hospital gown to get into and some plastic bags to put my clothes in. I was surprised when I discovered that my hospital gown was too small. I knew that my surgeon did many weight loss surgeries at this hospital and was surprised that they were not more prepared. I pointed out the small gown to a nurse and she immediately brought me a larger one. About 15 minutes after I went into the cubicle, my husband joined me. He kept me company while I waited for my trip to the operating room. Each of the cubicles had a television, so we were able to watch the early morning news. I was given an IV that was obviously a relaxant, because I was not nervous while I was waiting. Considering my hysteria during the last few days before my surgery, they must have given me a dose of something very good! My husband and I talked and joked while I lay in bed awaiting my 7:30 AM surgery appointment.

About 15 minutes before my surgery, the staff psychologist, Dr. Paul Friday, arrived. We had previously arranged for him to hypnotize me prior to surgery in an effort to promote healing and speed my recovery. He would also be with me during the surgery to mentally hold my hand by saying messages of relaxation and healing to me while I was being operated on. He had planned to arrive earlier than this, but as luck would have it, he got a speeding ticket that morning, which delayed him. As soon as the psychologist arrived, my anesthesiologist came in. He introduced himself and we all chatted about the procedure he was going to use to apply and monitor my anesthesia. He was concerned when he found out that I was being hypnotized, but warmed to the idea when I explained that the hypnosis was for relaxation and healing purposes only, and in no way was I expecting that I would receive less anesthesia.

The psychologist did not have a great deal of time to spend with me prior to my surgery but he was able to put me into a light trance. I do not remember going to the operating room or getting onto the operating table, so I know that the hypnosis did work. Unfortunately, I was awakened before my surgery by voices saying that my surgeon was delayed in traffic. I suddenly realized that my arms were strapped down and I could not breathe. I was having a panic attack. They decided to increase the anesthesia to sedate me, and just wait until my surgeon arrived. By this time, the psychologist had gotten into his scrubs for the surgery and was in the operating room with me. Throughout my surgery, he continued to say healing messages to me, reassuring me that my surgery would be successful. I was not conscious of his words, but I believe that his messages were effective.

I was hypnotized prior to surgery and my hypnotist repeated healing statements during surgery.

The next thing I remember was waking up in the operating room and looking up at my surgeon who told me that the surgery was over and that everything had gone well. The surgery had lasted about three hours. I knew that his wife just had a baby, so I asked him how the baby was. After he told me, I promptly fell back to sleep.

The next time I awoke, my eyes experienced the blinding bright lights of the recovery room. I hurt so badly and I wanted my husband. Every time I would ask where he was, I would be told only that my hospital room was not yet ready and I would fall back to sleep. Visitors were strictly prohibited from entering the recovery room. This went on for about four hours. At one point, because of my husband's insistence, he was allowed to visit me in the recovery room, but because of the drugs that were still in my system, I don't remember talking to him.

Finally, I was wheeled up to my room where my husband was waiting. He looked so wonderful to me. The love in his eyes alone helped to heal me. He had to step out for a few minutes while the nurse put me into my bed and checked my vital signs. When he came back in and I started to awaken further, I was told how to operate the morphine pump. I became very adept at pushing that button! But I still had pain despite the morphine, so I asked the nurse if the doctor had ordered anything additional for pain. He had and it was a drug called Toradol, which is a non-narcotic pain medication. When the dose of Toradol was injected into my IV line, I received instant relief. I continued to use the morphine pump regularly and periodically the nurse would inject another dose of Toradol. From that point on, the pain was quite manageable during the rest of my hospital stay.

I took my first "walk" a few hours after my surgery. I was expected to walk four or five times a day while in the hospital.

I took my first walk soon after that. The nurse instructed me on the easiest and least painful way to get out of bed. She told me to roll onto my right side and push myself up by putting my left arm against the mattress. It is easier than trying to use your stomach muscles to try to sit up. Getting out of all the attached paraphernalia is a bit tricky. I had to wear a massaging device on my legs to prevent blood clots, which had to be taken off every time I got out of bed. I also had to hang my catheter bag onto my IV pole so I could move around. My IV and morphine pump had to be disconnected from the wall plug and the cord wound up. The process was very cumbersome. It took both my husband and a nurse to steady me as I stood up because I felt very dizzy. The best I could do was to walk to the door of my room and back on that first attempt. It was certainly a lot of preparation for such a very short stroll. After I got back into bed, all of the equipment had to be reinstalled.

That evening, my family came to visit. Seeing my condition, they were kind enough to stay for only 30 minutes. I kept falling asleep, so they knew that I needed rest. We had previously made arrangements for my husband to remain with me during my hospital stay. I had a private room, and the hospital staff was able to provide him with a cot with sheets and a blanket. Although not as good as home, we were nice and cozy. I was not permitted to drink anything at that time, but I was allowed to wipe my mouth out with a small sponge on a stick that was dipped in ice chips. It was not enough liquid to affect anything, but it refreshed my mouth. I did not go to the bathroom that night. I was catheterized and grateful that I did not have to move. I was awakened several times during the night for normal checks of my vitals but I was able to quickly go back to sleep.

Post Surgery Days...

On my second day in the hospital, the staff worked to get me back to the many different ways to be "normal." Normal first means starting to walk again. I was to stroll around the hallways at least four times that day. It was exhausting, but I managed. Normal means breathing properly. I was given a device known as an incentive spirometer to help me breathe deeply. I was to exhale as much as possible, then inhale through the mouthpiece of this device to make a small ball go up to a certain point. This measures the amount of air that you take into your lungs and must be done periodically throughout the day. It is not only an indication of your current lung capacity, but is also a good exercise for your lungs. Normal means passing gas and having a bowel movement. I was able to accomplish this, but I could never figure out where everything was coming from. I was certainly empty after the Fleet Phospho Soda I took during my preparation for surgery and I had not eaten anything in four days. I guess it is one of those medical mysteries! I'm sorry for the blunt discussion about personal body functions, but these functions are absolutely vital to a good recovery. Normal also means that my new stomach did not leak. This was where I ran into some trouble.

Before noon on the day after my surgery, I was scheduled to have what is known as a "swallow" test. In this test, the patient drinks a barium liquid while being X-rayed, so that a radiologist can follow the path of the liquid to see if there are any leaks from the new pouch into the abdominal cavity. To my horror, I failed my swallow test when a tiny leak was suspected. As I was taken back up to my room, my mind was flooded with many terrible thoughts. I was very frightened and so grateful that my husband was there to comfort me.

14

Later that day, I spoke with my surgeon who explained the situation. He said that there probably wasn't a leak . The x-ray showed a spot that was interperted as a possible leak by the radiologist. Leaks are rare, but they do happen from time to time. In most cases, a leak will seal itself, but sometimes the surgeon has to go back in to repair it. Dr. Schauer instructed me to continue having nothing by mouth for the rest of the day so that another swallow test could be done on the following day. Since midnight prior to my surgery, my only source of hydration and medicine was the IV. On Thursday morning, I was taken to have another swallow test and this time the radiologist did not detect the spot that was noted on the first test. I was very excited about the test results and was looking forward to having my first liquid when I got back to my room. Not so!! For my safety, Dr. Schauer chose a very conservative approach. Being the conscientious doctor that he is, Dr. Schauer wanted the test done a third time to be absolutely sure that there was no leak. However, he did not want the third test done right away. If there was in fact a tiny leak that did seal, he did not want the test itself to exert extra pressure by having me drink the barium solution again so soon.

I was very disappointed to learn that he scheduled my next swallow test for a full week later!! That meant that I could have nothing by mouth for another whole week. As it turned out, I had to stay in the hospital for another two days because one of my lungs developed a condition know as atelectasis. This is literally collapsed air-sacs within the lung which is a fairly common, mild complication of surgery that resolves without special treatment. I also had a low-grade fever. Although these new problems were nothing terribly serious, they were enough to concern me.

Saturday arrived and I was finally going to be discharged. After my catheter was removed, my husband and I were trained on using IV therapy in the home. Since I still could not have anything by mouth for another week, I had to maintain my fluids and medication with an IV. Arrangements were made for a visiting nurse to set me up at home and answer any questions about how to administer the IV. My husband was responsible for changing the fluid bags and checking the IV pump for proper operation. About two hours before I was discharged, I was disconnected from my IV for the one-hour drive home and arrived at about 4:00 PM.

When the nurse arrived at about 5:00 PM, she proceeded to get my IV set up, but things did not go well. She could not find a good vein to get the IV started. She tried and tried, but she could not do it. She wrapped my arms in hot, wet towels hoping they would make my veins more visible. She tapped my arm where my veins should be, but found nothing! What you have to realize is that I now had been off the IV for about ten hours. Since I could not take anything by mouth, because I was dealing with a possible leak, my only ability to receiving life-giving fluids had failed!

At this point, my husband could not take any more of this floundering, and insisted that the nurse stop and immediately call her supervisor for help, which she did right away. In the meantime, Dr. Schauer called to see how I was doing, and hearing about the problems at home, said that if the nurses couldn't get the IV started, I would have to go back to the hospital.

Once I could shed my trailing IV and tubes, I felt like I was truly on my way. I had made it to the "Other Side."

About an hour later, at 10:00 PM, another nurse arrived who was an absolute angel. She looked at my wrist, found a vein, and got the IV started right away. What an expert! I will never forget her. She was not about to see me go back to the hospital. She had too much professional pride to see someone else do a job that she was perfectly capable of doing.

The next few days were uneventful. It was now over a week since I had any food or water by mouth. I think back and it seems like it should have been much worse than it was, but it really wasn't that bad. The worst part was not being able to take any pain medication.

I had to take morphine suppositories that were not strong enough. I could have used that liquid Roxicet that my surgeon had prescribed for pain!

Finally, the day of my third swallow test arrived! I passed with flying colors and was given the go ahead by Dr. Schauer to start my liquid diet. I immediately shed my IV's. How wonderful to have the freedom to move without trailing tubes. I went home and had a small bit of apple juice and have never tasted anything so good in my life!

I progressed slowly from that point. Because of abdominal pain, I couldn't stretch out comfortably in my bed, so I slept in a reclining chair for the next week. During the surgery, a tube was installed that stays in for ten days. The drain is called a Jackson Pratt drain and consists of a tube that went into one of my incisions, with a squeeze bottle on the end. This drain did not allow me to roll over onto my side and the recliner kept me in one position. It was terrific when I could finally sleep in my own bed again. I had come a long way in such a short amount of time since the surgery and was excited about the rest of my journey to a new thinner and healthier life.

3

Is Weight Loss Surgery For You?

You've been overweight all of your life. You were a chubby baby, were on diets when you were 12, and have always had a weight problem. You still have your baby fat. You go on diets, lose weight, but gain back more than you lost. You have first hand familiarity with Weight Watchers, the grapefruit diet, Jenny Craig, Nutri/System, the cabbage soup diet, the rotation diet, the high carbohydrate diet, Slim•Fast, the pineapple diet, the high fat diet, the Atkins diet, the Zone diet, and the list goes on and on. Does this sound like you? Well I know it sounds like me. I have even considered sending Christmas cards to Suzanne Powters, Suzanne Sommer, Mary Lou Henner and Fergie. Like me, you may have also tried amphetamines, the controversial Phen-Fen and Redux, Meridia or Xenical. Even though you are a self-made nutritional expert you still cannot control your weight.

We have lived with failure for so long that our self-esteem is nonexistent. Society does not understand what it is like to have a true weight problem. People who are not overweight look at us as being weak, and whisper or laugh behind our backs while they discriminate against us. They see an overweight person and think that losing weight is easy. What they do not understand is that obesity is a dreadful disease that for some reason we cannot control. Yet your doctor, family, and friends think that all you have to do is to exercise and eat less. They think it's simple. If they only knew how really hard it is.

But if it is so simple, then why is obesity at such epidemic proportions. The World Health Organization has declared that we are in the midst of a "global obesity epidemic." In a recent report, T. I. A. Sorensen, a scientist with the Institute of Preventive Medicine in Copenhagen, Denmark, commented on this epidemic as an overwhelming and growing problem. The current figures from the National Institutes of Health support this trend for the United States. Ninety-seven million American adults, or 55 percent, are in the overweight classification. Forty million American adults, or nearly 25 percent, are classified as obese. And one in ten children are considered to be overweight. In 1950 only one-quarter of Americans were classified as overweight. "The scales aren't lying...We have a serious weight problem," said Health and Human Services Secretary Donna Shalala. This is a huge understatement.

> *"If left untreated, patients who are morbidly obese have only a one in seven chance of reaching their life expectancy."*
> ***British Medical Journal***

Some have speculated that several million years of evolution is the culprit for our growing obesity dilemma. Our hunter-gatherer ancestors had to work constantly to provide food for themselves and their families so that evolution favored those who craved energy-rich fatty foods. And it looks like we will continue to get fatter. Dr. George Blackburn, of the Association for the Study of Obesity, has noted that in 1975, 25 percent of women were overweight. Currently 51 percent of women are overweight. And in 2025, the percentage of overweight women is expected to increase to 75 percent of women. Further, currently 6 percent of women and 2 percent of men are morbidly obese.

Studies have shown that people are genetically predisposed to morbid obesity. Adopted children follow the body type of their birth parents rather than that of their adoptive parents who provide them with an environment and teach them nutrition. Identical twins who share the same genes have much more similar body types than fraternal twins who do not share the same genes.

Whatever the reason, and regardless of how much company you have, you may have reached the point at which you are no longer able to live with your obesity. But are you willing to take the step to have weight loss surgery? Weight loss surgery is a life-altering, permanent and major step, not without its risks. However, living with obesity is also very risky. The mortality rate in weight loss surgery is less than one percent, about the same as having any other surgery. Yet those who are morbidly obese can expect a 15 year shorter life span, with a quality of life that is often affected by difficulty breathing, high blood pressure, severe joint pain, diabetes, heart problems, increased risk of breast cancer, inability to become pregnant, depression, and a life that is also affected by discrimination and derision.

Weight loss surgery is not without its risks.
However, living with obesity is also risky.

After giving you the facts about the obesity problem in the world, we come again to the main question that started this section. Is weight loss surgery for you? Very simply, you must evaluate your life as it is today with your current weight, and factor in your rate of weight gain each year for the rest of your life. Subtract several years off your life span for increasing medical problems and consider the declining quality of life for your remaining years. After doing this, consider the fact that you have a procedure available that can help you to reverse all your weight problems and actually allow you to become thin. I did all of these calculations and considerations and came to the conclusion that gastric bypass surgery was definitely for me. The result of this decision has allowed me to lose well over 125 pounds of life draining weight and has given me a quality of life that I never thought was possible again. When you look at the decision as a balance between having surgery or continuing your life as it is today (and what it will become in the future), the choice is obvious.

4
Diets Vs Surgery:
How Successful Can I Expect to Be?

Successful weight loss is an unattainable goal for most people. Despite the fact that we spend $33 billion dollars annually trying to lose weight, the problem is that common methods like diets and exercise plans simply do not work. It is estimated that 95 percent of all people who have dieted will regain the weight that they lost within three years and most will actually be heavier then when they started. The National Institutes of Health Technology Assessment Panel concluded that weight reduction programs have been a dismal failure for the morbidly obese and that diet medications result in only a loss of 6 to 10 percent of weight. But you probably already know this from your own experience in trying to control your own weight. In contrast, the periodical <u>Obesity Surgery</u> in its April 1997 issue reported a 4-year study of proximal Roux en-Y (RNY) gastric bypass patients. The table below shows the average excess weight lost during this study.

Years Post-Op	Percent Excess Weight Lost
1	68.5 percent
2	71.18 percent
3	69.28 percent
4	57.49 percent

What this table shows is that a 5'6" woman who weighs 260 pounds can expect to lose 83.5 pounds the first year following weight loss surgery. This is the average. Some will lose more and some will lose less. In my own case, I lost that amount of weight in just six months. The study also found that the average patient is a 40-year old with a pre-surgery weight of about 325 pounds. Eighty percent of the approximately 45,000 weight loss surgeries that are done each year are done on women.

The National Institutes of Health, at their 1992 conference, concluded that non-surgical methods of losing weight do not work in the long term for those who are severely obese. ***Weight loss surgery works***. It is a tool that can change your life by allowing you to lose massive amounts of weight. It is the only treatment found to be effective for morbid obesity. If you want to lose weight for the long term, don't look to the standard everyday methods. Diets don't work; drugs don't work; exercise and behavior modification don't work, for the long-term. And that is the problem. We are all experts at losing pounds in the short term, but it all comes back in the long term.

Many people are concerned that when they have dieted in the past, they have felt nervous, weak, hungry, obsessed with food, tired and generally not good. They wonder if that is the way they will feel after surgery. The answer is a resounding, "no!" There are times of hunger, especially in the beginning when you are experiencing "head hunger." This is hunger that doesn't really exist. It is the time when your body is expecting to be fed at the same times it was fed in the past. This soon subsides because your body goes through a behavior modification process that is physically imposed by the surgery. The first 12 to 18 months after surgery is known as the "Window of Opportunity." When you eat or drink anything during this window, you soon discover that a very small amount fills you up. When you try to eat more than your capacity, you will feel ill and throw up. When you do this enough times, you become turned off to food. This window provides you with an effective tool to lose a large amount of weight early on. After your window has closed and you have lost most of your weight, you will be able to eat and drink a slightly larger amount. Feelings of true hunger also return, but never to the extent that existed before the surgery.

I knew that every pound I lost was gone forever.
Finally, I won the weight loss game.

How successful can you expect to be with weight loss surgery? You can expect to be far more successful than with conventional dieting methods. But remember that success should be measured in more than weight loss. Rejoice in the first time that you can cross your legs, or fit comfortably in the bath tub with a little bit of room to spare. Success is getting off of your blood pressure medication or walking your first mile without huffing and puffing. Success is going to an amusement park and having the bar go down on a ride. Success is fitting in a lawn chair or not having to use an extension seat belt on an airplane. Success is the first time that you can shop in a regular clothes department instead of the plus size department, or the first time that you can paint your toenails. Success is the satisfaction that you have lost a tremendous amount of excess weight and you know that it will *never* come back.

5
Do You Qualify For Surgery?

The National Institutes of Health established the following guidelines for considering patients for weight loss surgery. Patients should:
> ➤ Be at least 100 pounds overweight
> ➤ Should have a co-morbidity that will be improved by the surgery
> ➤ Should be intelligent enough to understand the surgery and risks
> ➤ Should have no glandular problems causing their obesity
> ➤ Should have tried to lose weight by conventional means
> ➤ Should be willing to be observed over a long period of time.

Surgeons are not regulated by these guidelines but most will use them to determine eligibility of prospective patients.

1) Pounds Overweight - Your BMI

Most surgeons and insurance companies consider your Body Mass Index (BMI) to determine your eligibility for weight loss surgery. BMI is calculated by dividing your weight by your height squared.

The following is a chart of BMI levels:

Underweight   < 18.5
Normal 18.5-24.9
Overweight   25-29.9
Obese I 30-34.9
Obese II   35-39.9
Morbidly Obese   >40

A BMI of 40 or above is considered a qualification for weight loss surgery. Often, a BMI of just 35 or above with co-morbidities is also considered justification. In addition to considering your BMI, most insurance companies and some doctors require that you be 100 or more pounds overweight according to the Metropolitan Life Insurance height and weight charts. Refer to the chart below to determine your own BMI.

Height In inches	40	41	42	43	44	45	46	47	48	49	50	51	52	53	54	55	56	57	58	59	60
									Body Mass Index (BMI) Value												
58	191	196	201	206	211	215	221	225	230	234	239	244	249	254	258	263	265	273	278	283	287
59	198	203	208	213	218	223	228	233	238	243	248	253	257	262	267	272	277	282	287	292	297
60	205	210	215	220	225	230	236	241	246	251	256	261	266	271	276	282	287	292	297	302	307
61	212	217	222	228	233	238	243	249	254	259	265	270	275	281	286	291	296	302	307	312	318
62	219	224	230	235	241	246	252	257	262	268	273	279	284	290	295	301	306	312	317	323	328
63	226	232	237	243	248	254	260	265	271	277	282	288	294	299	305	311	316	322	327	333	339
64	233	239	245	251	256	262	268	274	280	286	292	297	303	309	315	321	326	332	338	344	350
65	240	246	252	258	264	270	277	283	289	295	301	307	313	319	325	331	337	343	349	355	361
66	248	254	260	266	273	279	285	291	298	304	310	316	322	328	335	341	347	353	359	366	372
67	255	262	268	275	281	287	294	300	307	313	319	326	332	338	345	351	358	364	370	377	383
68	263	270	276	283	290	296	303	309	316	322	329	336	342	349	355	362	368	375	382	388	395
69	271	278	285	291	298	305	312	318	325	332	339	346	352	359	366	373	379	386	393	400	406
70	279	286	293	300	307	314	321	328	335	342	349	356	363	370	377	383	390	397	404	411	418
71	287	294	301	309	316	323	330	337	344	352	359	366	373	380	387	395	402	409	416	423	430
72	295	303	310	317	325	332	339	347	354	362	369	376	384	391	398	406	413	421	428	435	443

Body Mass Index (BMI) Chart

Locate your height in the left column. Scan right to find your weight. Then scan to top to determine your BMI value.

2) Should have a co-morbidity that will be improved by the surgery.

Co-morbidities are those conditions that are caused by or affected by excessive weight. This consideration of weight loss surgery will be discussed more thoroughly in Chapter 6.

3) Should be intelligent enough to understand the surgery and its risks.

There should be no doubt about the fact that weight loss surgery is a very major operation that will have a profound impact on the patient for the rest of his or her life. This fact cannot be overstated. The procedure involves making the stomach smaller and rerouting the intestinal tract to create a limited ability to eat normal amounts of food. Gastric bypass surgery is reversible, but because the surgery is so successful, it is an extreme rarity that patients want to go back to the way they were before.

Weight loss surgery is not without its risks. The American Society for Bariatric Surgery reports that the mortality rate within 30 days of surgery is 0.17 percent. This means that out of 1,000 morbidly obese people who have this surgery, less than 2 die within 30 days of surgery. This is very low, but of course not if you are the one that died! But if you consider that people having this surgery are very high-risk patients, then the rate is particularly low. Many are told by their doctors that if they don't have this surgery, they will die very soon. Taking this into consideration, weight loss surgery is as safe as any other surgery.

It is important that you understand the risks associated with this surgery. Do your research and discuss this with your surgeon.

However being obese is also risky. A study done in 1979 published in the <u>Journal of Chronic Diseases</u> following 750,000 people showed that people who are obese or 50 percent overweight are twice as likely to die than those of normal weight. The mortality rate for diabetics is even worse. Men who are diabetic are five times more likely to die prematurely and woman who are diabetic are eight times as likely to die prematurely as those who are not obese.

Those who are morbidly obese, with a Body Mass Index of 40 or above (or more than 100 pounds overweight) are at a far greater risk. There is an ongoing Swedish Study that is following 2,000 morbidly obese patients. Half of the study group is the "diet" group and the other half is the "surgery" group. During the 6 years of the study, 3 people in the surgery group died while 27 people in the diet group died, showing a 9 times difference in mortality. Weight loss surgery can not only improve your life, but can also save your life.

4) Should have no glandular problems causing their obesity.

Many of us have at one time believed that our weight problem had to be glands. It couldn't be that we over ate!! But only a very small fraction of those who are obese, are so because of glandular problems. According to originator of the Fobi Pouch, Dr. Mathias Fobi, only 2 percent of the morbidly obese have a glandular problem that causes people to become overweight. In preparing for surgery, most of us go through extensive tests to determine our general health. At that time, if any glandular problems are found that could cause obesity, they can be addressed before surgery is pursued.

5) Should have tried to lose weight by conventional means

Gain weight, lose weight, gain more weight, lose weight, and gain even more weight.... Does this sound familiar? The cycle of yo-yo dieting is well known to each of us. And although diets are not effective for those who are morbidly obese, you are expected to have made an attempt to lose weight the traditional way through diet and exercise. Unfortunately, a few insurance companies use this recommendation from the National Institutes of Health to insist that each person who is approved first go through the insurance company's own dieting program, adding yet another failure to an already damaged ego.

6) Should be willing to be observed over a long period of time

Weight loss surgery has been performed since 1954. Since that time, many studies have revealed potential long-term side effects that patients are prone to. These include such problems as nutritional deficiencies and bowel obstructions from growing adhesions. Your surgeon will know what to look for during your follow-up exams and will check your blood levels to determine any deficiencies. Weight loss surgery alters you in a major way. It is a serious undertaking and you will need to be followed by a medical professional to ensure that you retain your newly found good health as the years go by.

6
Co-Morbidities

Co-morbidities are those conditions that are caused by or affected by excessive weight. These would include joint pain, diabetes, sleep apnea, heart condition, reflux esophagitis, certain types of cancer, depression, difficulty breathing, a rash from excessive skin or thighs rubbing, incontinence, and inability to get pregnant. The Alvarado Center for Surgical Weight Control reports that 95 percent of all co-morbidities are relieved within 1 year after surgery. Many surgeons and insurance companies will consider you to be eligible for surgery with a BMI of 35 with co-morbidities or a BMI of 40 with no co-morbidities.

Here are some of the more common health problems created by obesity that can be classified as co-morbidities. This list of co-morbidities is not all-inclusive. The key to determine if a specific problem can be classified as a co-morbidity is to consider how being overweight affects the condition.

Morbid Obesity And The Heart

The larger a body is, the more volume of blood that must be circulated through it. With more blood to pump, the heart must work harder, even when a person is at rest. The heart is a muscle, and as the heart works harder, this muscle gets thicker. This thickening affects the contraction of the heart and its relaxation. Over time, the heart may not be able to keep up with the increased load. The result may be congestive heart failure with shortness of breath. Angina, or chest pain, is caused by a decrease of oxygen to the heart. High levels of blood fats, cholesterol and triglycerides, can also lead to heart disease. These are all linked to obesity. The American Heart Association has found that obese adults are three times more likely to develop hypertension than those who are not obese. Those who are morbidly obese are six times more likely to develop heart disease.

As weight increases, so does blood pressure. Elevated blood pressure, or hypertension, leads to heart disease, blood vessel damage and susceptibility to strokes, kidney damage and hardening of the arteries. Studies have shown that the more weight lost by obese patients, the more improvement there is to heart abnormalities.

The direct and indirect health care costs of heart disease related to obesity are $7 billion dollars annually.

Morbid Obesity and Diabetes

Non-insulin dependent diabetes mellitus (type 2 diabetes) is the most common diabetes in the United States. It reduces your ability to control your blood sugar and is a major cause of heart disease, stroke, kidney disease and blindness. Obesity is a major cause of diabetes, and those who are obese are ten times more likely to develop diabetes. Diabetes is the leading cause of adult-onset blindness and the major cause of kidney failure

A 14-year study that appeared in the journal, <u>Annals of Surgery</u> in 1995 found that the best therapy for diabetes is weight loss surgery. This study followed 608 morbidly obese patients with diabetes who underwent gastric bypass surgery. The mean weight before surgery was 304 pounds. One year after surgery, the mean weight was 192 pounds. The patients were able to maintain their weight at approximately 205 pounds for 14 years. Over the 14-year period, between 83 percent and 99 percent of patients maintained normal glucose and insulin levels. The study goes on to say that gastric bypass surgery is now established as an effective and safe therapy for morbid obesity and its associated morbidities. No other therapy has produced such durable and complete control of diabetes mellitus. That is an incredible endorsement. However the surgery did not do all the work. What it did was to allow patients to control their eating habits, which in turn resulted in rapid weight loss that enabled them to control their diabetes.

In a 1996 study done by Dr. K.C. MacDonald at the East Carolina University School of Medicine in Greenville, NC, 154 obese Non-Insulin Dependent Diabetes Mellitus (NIDDM) patients who had undergone gastric bypass surgery were compared to a group of NIDDM patients who had not undergone surgery. The study found that 82 percent of the non-surgical patients required anti-diabetic medication as opposed to only 7 percent of the surgical patients. Also of significance was that the patients who did not have surgery had a 4 1/2 times greater mortality rate than those that did have surgery. The study showed gastric bypass surgery not only greatly improved the quality of life of obese diabetic patients, but the surgery also saved lives.

Diabetes is the number three cause of death in the United States. The direct and indirect annual cost of type II diabetes related to obesity is $63 billion.

Morbid Obesity and Sleep Apnea

Because morbidly obese people have a large abdomen, when they lie down to sleep, they may notice a shortness of breath as the abdomen interferes with the function of the diaphragm. When lying down, gravity exerts pressure on the thickened tissues and muscles of the throat and neck. This causes a restriction that blocks the flow of air to the lungs that interrupts the breathing process, a condition called apnea. Because there is less air going into the lungs, apnea reduces the amount of oxygen in the blood. Low oxygen due to apnea can affect the rhythm of the heart and may be responsible for some cases of sudden death during sleep, accumulation of carbon dioxide in the blood, and heart failure. Waking frequently during the night causes sleep apnea patients to feel sleepy during the day and may lead them to fall asleep while driving.

Morbid Obesity and Cancer

Several types of cancer are associated with obesity. For women, these include cancer of the uterus, gall bladder, cervix, ovary, breast and colon. Obese men are at a greater risk of developing prostate, colon and rectal cancer. Approximately 42 percent of colon cancer occurs in obese patients.

Morbid Obesity and Osteoarthritis

Osteoarthritis is a common joint disease that affects the joints in the knees, hips and lower back. As your weight increases, excessive pressure is put on these joints causing the cartilage that cushions these joints to squeeze out or wear away much faster than in normal weighted persons.

Morbid Obesity and Respiratory Problems

People who are obese or morbidly obese often find that they have difficulty breathing. The wall of the chest is very heavy and difficult to lift during normal respiration, and because of a large body size, the need for oxygen is greater. They become very short of breath during regular activity. Sometimes there will be toxic levels of carbon dioxide in the blood. This lack of oxygen is not only tiring, but also disabling when the person is not able to function normally.

Morbid Obesity, Heartburn, and Reflux Disease

When stomach acid escapes through the valve at the top of the stomach up into the esophagus, heartburn or acid indigestion results. When this happens during sleep, the acid may be inhaled, searing the airway. There is also the possibility of pneumonia or injury to the lungs. In the extreme state, this reflux can lead to cancer of the esophagus. Many obese people suffer from reflux disease.

Morbid Obesity and Gall Bladder Disease

Repeated attempts to lose weight followed by regaining weight often leads to the formation of gallstones as bile becomes saturated with cholesterol. When these cause pain or a disease of the gall bladder, the gall bladder must be removed. Often the gall bladder is removed during weight loss surgery.

Morbid Obesity and Stress Urinary Incontinence

A large abdomen and relaxed pelvic muscles from childbirth may cause the valve on the urinary bladder to weaken. This causes leakage of urine when you cough, sneeze or laugh. This condition is associated with obesity and is relieved by weight loss.

Morbid Obesity and Depression

Those who are morbidly obese face many social and emotional issues. They have dealt with feelings of failure all their lives as they have tried repeatedly to control something that is beyond their control. The result of the dieter's failure is always very visible because it is right out there for everyone to see. I know when I have gone on diets and lost a lot of weight, everyone was so complimentary about my weight loss. Then as I started to regain that weight, no one said a word. Yet I knew what they were thinking, and it was the same as I was thinking, that I couldn't stop myself from eating. If I just could leave that food alone I wouldn't be so fat. How could I be so undisciplined? When you add to these feelings of failure and its accompanying low self esteem, the social stigma and discrimination that we endure, is it any wonder that this leads to depression?

Morbid Obesity and Pregnancy

Many morbidly obese women find that they are unable to conceive. This occasionally results from the fact that estrogen is stored in and converted by fat cells. When a woman's body has too much (or too little) fat, the normal menstrual cycle is interrupted or stopped. Several studies have shown that soon after weight loss surgery, ovulation starts again, followed by spotting and regular periods.

Those morbidly obese women who do become pregnant are often considered high-risk pregnancies because of the co-morbidities that are often present such as high blood pressure and diabetes. Therefore, even when the morbidly obese woman achieves pregnancy, carrying the pregnancy to full-term is very risky.

7
Insurance Coverage

Weight loss surgery is a major procedure. The cost of surgery can vary greatly, with laparoscopic RNY surgery being the most expensive, costing up to $60,000 although the average cost is approximately $15,000 to $20,000. Since the surgery is a medical necessity, sometimes required to save your life, your insurance company should be paying for it. Depending upon your insurance company and how your plan is written, getting insurance coverage can be either extremely easy or it can be a struggle. If you meet the National Institutes of Health (NIH) minimum guidelines of being at least 100 pounds overweight, with a BMI of 40 or over with any co-morbidities at all, and have been unsuccessful at losing weight through dieting, then you should be successful in getting your surgery covered. If your particular insurance plan excludes weight loss surgery, you could be in for a major battle. But even if that exclusion does exist in your plan, it can still be possible for the surgery to be covered. I will cover how this is done later in this chapter.

Weight loss surgery is becoming so common and successful that the States of Georgia and Virginia have passed legislation that directs employers and insurance companies to provide coverage for weight loss surgery as an option to employees. The law provides that as long as employees meet National Institutes of Health guidelines for surgery eligibility, applications for this benefit should not be denied.

Here are some steps that you can take to assure insurance coverage.

Start With Your Primary Care Physician

Getting insurance coverage is a lot smoother if you can have your primary care physician (PCP) refer you to a surgeon. More of your surgery will be paid for and your insurance company will look more favorably on your request for coverage. Your PCP is in possession of your medical history that you will need to develop your case to the insurance company. Your physician also is probably familiar with your weight struggles over the years and will be able to attest to the fact that common diets haven't worked for you. Often however, PCP's aren't informed about the latest techniques in weight loss surgery and only know about older, more dangerous procedures known for their severe complications. Therefore they may have a prejudice against the surgery. If you are convinced that you will benefit from this surgery, do not let your PCP dissuade you because he or she is misinformed. You may want to educate your physician by getting together a packet of research material on weight loss surgery and include a copy of this book. But if your PCP will not refer you, and from your research you are convinced that you will benefit from weight loss surgery, then get a new PCP.

There are several ways to find a new primary care physician. First, find out if your insurance coverage requires you to select a PCP from a specified network of doctors or if you have unrestricted selection. Then call several doctors in your area and ask the nurse if the doctor does referrals for weight loss surgery. Another thing you can do is to contact a surgeon who performs weight loss surgery and ask what PCPs refer to him or her.

My own PCP did refer me, but I was very nervous about asking. I was dealing with my own feelings of failure at the time. Very reluctantly, he had prescribed Phen-Fen for me years earlier. I of course lost weight, but regained it when I had to go off the medication when national alerts were issued about the health problems arising from the medication. He then referred me to a nutritional physician who worked with me on a behavior modification plan combined with Meridia. That worked also, but again I regained the weight. And here I was asking for yet another weight loss solution. I wanted this surgery so badly and feared that he would deny me. But to my surprise and joy, he did refer me, which made my journey easier.

Documentation

On one of your initial visits to your surgeon, you should receive a packet of forms for you to provide background information. The surgeon will be interested in knowing if there is a history of obesity in your family and what co-morbidities you have (high blood pressure, respiratory problems, joint pain, diabetes, sleep apnea, heart problems, skin rashes caused by excess skin, depression, incontinence, inability to get pregnant, etc.). The surgeon will also want to know about your attempts to lose weight through dieting, behavior modification classes, or medication and how you have regained weight after those losses. Also of interest is what social, psychological and economical effect your obesity has had on your life. It is important that you be as detailed as possible when filling out these forms because this is the information that the surgeon uses to convince your insurance company that weight loss surgery is medically necessary. The more information that you can provide, the better off you are. If you do not receive a formal questionnaire from your surgeon, be prepared to give all of the above information when the surgeon questions you on subsequent visits. It is absolutely vital that you be able to answer all questions accurately and completely.

A brief letter from your primary care physician indicating support for your weight loss surgery can be very helpful. Also of great value are letters from any medical professionals who have treated you for health-related conditions caused by, or aggravated by, obesity. Do not be shy about asking for these letters because without them, your attempts to get insurance approval will be jeopardized. Request that the letters be sent directly to you so that if they are not completely supportive, then you do not have to use them. The more letters of support you have from medical professionals the better.

About a week after your surgeon's office staff has submitted all your forms and letters to the insurance company, double check with the insurance company that they have in fact received the information packet. This entire process can be very frustrating when the insurance company denies receiving anything. Call your surgeon's office and find out if and when they sent the packet. This is one time when being the "squeaky wheel" definitely pays off. Keep calling until the insurance company has the paperwork or admits to having it. Always keep track of whom you spoke to at the insurance company and your doctor's office along with the date and time you spoke with them.

Do not let weeks go by waiting for a verdict from the insurance company only to discover that they have no paperwork at all.

After receipt of the standard forms from your surgeon, some insurance companies will want additional proof that you have dieted and failed. In these cases, your primary care physician's notes of your weight history and any prescribed medication will help. Any receipts that you may have for weight loss medication or diet supplements can be copied and submitted. A copy of a Weight Watchers record book can be used. You can also submit pictures showing you at various weights when you have dieted and regained weight over the years.

My insurance company was Blue Cross/ Blue Shield Select Blue. Along with a BMI of 41, the only co-morbidity I had was severe joint and back pain. I was afraid that I was not "bad enough" to be approved. At this point, I was still in denial that I was really eligible for this surgery. However, I was approved in one day. When I got the news, I was so happy I cried. I was flooded with a feeling of relief and felt a validation of myself that I was not a total failure. The system acknowledged that my obesity was not a horrible weakness, or character flaw and was not my fault. It was a medical condition that was recognized by the medical and insurance community. It also became very real to me that I was actually going to have this surgery.

What If You Are Denied?

The surgeon's staff normally submits all of the paperwork to your insurance company for approval. Their submission is based upon the information that you provided prior to or at your first visit. Normally, they have a great deal of experience doing this, and do it quite well. However, some offices do it better than others. Ultimately however, insurance coverage is your responsibility, so you need to be proactive.

Some insurance companies will automatically deny weight loss surgery even if it is medically necessary. If you are denied, do not despair because it is not necessarily the final answer. Many people are approved after providing additional information. Some insurance companies will just say "no," while others will ask you endlessly for additional information, perhaps hoping that you will give up and just go away. Only 30% of patients fight back and many insurance companies count on this. If this surgery is what you want, don't give up. If they keep asking, keep giving them the information they want. Let the insurance company be the one who gives up and grants you approval.

If you meet the criteria for weight loss surgery set by the NIH, your insurance should cover this surgery. If you are denied, keep trying. Don't give up. You will be giving up on yourself.

Appealing

If you are denied coverage, you will have to write an appeal letter to your insurance company. I have included an example of an appeal letter as Appendix C to this book. You will want to include the following: State your name, height and weight. You should state your Body Mass Index (BMI), explain what a BMI is and how your BMI classifies you in terms of obesity. Discuss in your letter how long you have been overweight and indicate all diets you have been on. What effects have these diets had on you? What outcomes have you had from dieting, including weight loss and weight regain? What medications have you taken to try to lose weight? Have you been able to exercise, and how this affects you? List all of your co-morbidities.

38

The more you list, the more chance that your appeal will be successful. Do you have high blood pressure, sleep apnea, diabetes, degenerative joint disease, joint or back pain, swelling or numbness in your feet or limbs, incontinence, infertility, cardiovascular disease or gastro-esophageal reflux. If so, how do these affect you? Describe your family history as it relates to obesity. Are your parents or siblings obese? And if so, what co-morbidities are caused by their obesity? What medication do you normally take, including prescription medication and over-the-counter? How has your obesity caused or worsened co-morbidities? What social effect has your weight had on your life? Are you short of breath when you walk or climb a flight of stairs? Do you have difficulty completing normal daily routines such as shopping, cleaning, getting out of chairs, etc? Have you suffered any job related problems including difficulty moving about at work or loss of promotion because of your size? Do you suffer any depression because of your obesity? Also, state that you understand the benefits as well as the risks of this surgery. You may want to list both the benefits and the risks so it is very apparent that you know what they are.

In your appeal, emphasize how the surgery will relieve your co-morbidities. You are more inclined to win approval based on that approach, rather than the fact that you just want to lose weight.

This entire process can be very painful because it reminds you of the many times you have failed. However, if you remember that all of this is evidence that you have a medical condition that should be covered by your insurance company and not a failure on your part, it can be a bit easier.

Insurance companies count on the fact that people change insurance coverage about every three years. So an argument that you will cost your insurance company a lot of money in claims in the future will probably not be effective. They will reason that you will probably not be a member of their plan when that happens.

Insurance policy coverage is determined for the most part by whoever pays the premium, which is your employer. If your direct appeal to the insurance company is unsuccessful, you may want to appeal to your Human Relations Department where you or your spouse works. Discuss the situation with them. They may go to bat for you with the insurance company. If you are organized, you may want to start with your union representative rather than the Human Relations Department. Be prepared to defend your position with research material on the medical cost of morbid obesity and statistics on the success of weight loss surgery. This is especially important if you are dealing with a Director of Human Relations or Union Shop Steward who knew someone who had their stomach stapled ten years ago and regained all of their weight. You know the old story!

Much of the research material to defend your position is included or addressed in this book. Also, on my website, **http://www.wlscenter.com**, there is an extensive section of research material that can be printed out and presented as an information packet to the insurance company, your Human Relations Department, or your Union Representative.

If your appeal is not successful, you may want to consider hiring Walter Lindstrom to handle your appeal. Walter Lindstrom is an attorney in Chula Vista, California who has a law practice specializing in taking on insurance companies that refuse to cover the cost of weight loss surgery. Since Mr. Lindstrom has had weight loss surgery himself, he has first-hand knowledge of the medical necessity of the surgery as well as the legal aspects of insurance claims. While he rarely meets personally with clients, he normally conducts his business over the phone, fax or by mail, with clients from all over the country. He has a very good reputation in the weight loss surgery community and might be an avenue you want to pursue. His web site is **http://www.obesitylaw.com**.

If denied, because of limitations of ERISA (Employee Retirement Income Security Act of 1974) under which your company plan is regulated, you are actually better off if you have your own policy rather than one supplied by your employer.

Your Policy

If you are denied, begin by asking for a copy of your entire policy. You are entitled to more than just a short description in column format that most employers provide. Request the long form. Also ask for the Summary Plan Description for additional information.

Learn how to read your policy. Most policies will include the following sections:

> ➤ How the Policy Operates - Usually describes if you must select physicians from a network, 2nd opinions, testing, pre-certification, etc.

> ➤ Enrollment - Includes how to become a member and general enrollment information.

> ➤ Details of the Plan - Could include such information as what your PCP is responsible for, referrals, authorizations, and maximum payments.

> ➤ Grievance Procedure and Arbitration - This section will be important to you if your claim is denied. This section will detail the steps you will have to go through to appeal. Make good use of your appeal procedure. If you think there might be any chance at all of using an attorney, don't use up all of your appeal steps yourself. Save at least one for your attorney.

> ➤ Benefits - This is the most important section for you. Here you will find what is covered and what is not. Pay particular attention to this section. Remember that most policies will say that they do not cover treatment for weight loss and obesity. However, weight loss **surgery** is treatment for **morbid** obesity. That exclusion does not apply, unless it mentions a particular exclusion for weight loss surgery and morbid obesity. This section may also include details of hospital care, emergency services, and prescription medications.

➤ Other Sections: There may be sections on definitions, limitations and exclusions. These tend to be more general in nature, although the definitions sections might provide you with some helpful language.

Policies are difficult to comprehend, so reading and re-reading will be necessary. An excellent resource is the book Making Them Pay: How to Get the Most from Health Insurance and Managed Care by Rhonda Orin. It will help you to understand the maze of the insurance industry.

Support Group

Go to your local support group and stand up and ask if anyone has insurance coverage from XYZ Insurance Company. Consult with those people and find out if they had any trouble, how problems were resolved and if they spoke to anyone at XYZ who was particularly helpful. Find out if there is an OSSG group that covers your local area or State and ask the same questions.

Switch Insurance Companies

You also have the option of switching insurance companies. Often your employer will offer a choice of insurance companies. There is also the option of purchasing your own insurance. There are two points to remember in this process. Make sure that the insurance company that you are switching to covers weight loss surgery and that the plan you are going into includes weight loss surgery. Also remember that if you are new to a company they might not cover this surgery for the first year because they consider it a pre-existing condition. This is certainly preferable to paying for the surgery yourself, however any delay is a disappointment.

Self-Pay

You do have the option of paying for the surgery yourself if you have no insurance coverage or if you have exhausted all insurance avenues and appeals. I know of many people who have done this, but it was not an option that I would have wanted to try. My concern was not just the cost of the surgery, but also the question of possible complications necessitating additional surgery or a lengthier hospital stay. I could see financial ruin at the end of that scenario. Some surgeons will not perform weight loss surgery if you do not have insurance for just this reason.

But if you do proceed this way, try to negotiate a rate with your surgeon, hospital and anesthesiologist. You should not pay full fare. Try to pay the same amount that the insurance company would pay. That cost is usually a fraction of the billed cost. Sometimes the surgeon will set up a payment schedule for you. The cost can vary greatly from $15,000 to $60,000. Laparoscopic surgery is the most expensive because of the equipment involved and the special training of the staff.

Vocational Rehabilitation

Many States have a Department of Vocational or Occupational Rehabilitation and patients have had some success here. If you are unemployed and can convince the department that your morbid obesity has led to your inability to work, some States have funded the surgery. It is not an easy route, but is another avenue to try. You will need to be very aggressive and expect to hear that they don't cover it. You may be their first request. It has been covered at least in Texas and Arkansas. Check the telephone book for your local office.

8
Weight Loss Surgery:
A Brief Overview

The Digestive Process

In order to understand how weight loss surgery works, it is important that you understand how the normal digestive process occurs.

Digestion starts in our mouths as we chew our food and mix it with saliva. We swallow our food and it goes down our esophagus into our stomachs where food is stored for a period of time. A normal stomach is about the size of your head and holds about six cups of food. In the stomach, strong gastric juices mix with the food and continue the digestive process. The food then moves into the duodenum, the first part of the small intestines where bile and pancreatic juice speed up digestion. Digestion of meat and other protein occurs here and most of the iron and calcium from the food that we eat is absorbed in this part of the small intestines. The remaining two segments of the small intestines, the jejunum and ileum, complete the absorption of almost all calories and nutrients. What is not digested and absorbed in the nearly 20 feet of the small intestines is stored in the large intestines, or colon, until it can be eliminated.

History of Weight Loss Surgery

There are several types of weight loss surgery available today and all are classified as "bariatric surgery." Bariatric surgery has been performed in the United States for more than 20 years. The word "bariatric" is from the Greek word "baros" meaning weight and the Greek word "iatrike" meaning treatment. Bariatric surgery has been recognized as a surgical sub-specialty by the American College of Surgeons since 1982. But it was not until 1991, that a panel of experts from the National Institutes of Health endorsed this surgery as an effective method of weight reduction.

The concept of weight loss surgery as a treatment for obesity grew out of operations for cancer or severe ulcers in which large portions of the stomach or small intestines were removed. It was found that people having this surgery lost large amounts of weight. Surgeons then began to use such operations on the severely obese and found them to be very effective.

There are two types of surgeries that are currently endorsed by the National Institutes of Health. They are the Roux en-Y (RNY) gastric bypass surgery and the Vertical Banded Gastroplasty (VBG). I will devote a chapter to each of these surgeries.

Eighty percent of the weight loss surgeries performed every year are the RNY.

As in any science, early medical research and study of weight loss surgery has allowed procedures to evolve into the safe and effective surgeries we have today. Although these current surgeries have proven themselves by the thousands of successful operations performed each year, many people still hang on to past perceptions because of a lack of knowledge. The two early procedures presented below were critical in the evolution of weight loss surgery, but were discontinued due to the problems discovered. Many people (including some primary care physicians) who claim to know about weight loss surgery only have a faint knowledge about these past procedures.

Jejuno-ileal Bypass

This surgery was first done in 1954 and was the first attempt at surgically induced weight loss. This procedure was a malabsorption procedure, bypassing most of the small intestines. The idea was that patients could eat large amounts of food, which would be poorly digested or passed along so fast that the body could not absorb the calories. Many complications were associated with this surgery including a loss of essential nutrients, severe diarrhea, kidney stones, electrolyte imbalances, liver failure, and death. This surgery is no longer being performed in the United States.

Although this surgery has not been performed since about 1982, many people associate weight loss surgery with the jejuno-ileal bypass. They incorrectly assume that the surgery being performed today carries the same risk, complications, and mortality rate. This is far from correct.

Gastroplasty

This surgery is commonly known as "stomach stapling" and is usually what comes to mind when discussing weight loss surgery today. It was developed in 1979 at Ohio State University. There were many variations of this surgery, but the most common involved placing a row of staples horizontally all the way across the upper part of the stomach, and removing three staples in the middle of the row. This allowed food to pass slowly from the upper stomach to the lower stomach. Although the surgery was initially successful, the small pouch would tend to stretch or the staples would work loose and the patient would regain all of the lost weight. Because of a common failure of the staple line, this surgery has mostly been abandoned.

Many people confuse the former stomach stapling with the successful modern procedures that are done today.

46

9
Choosing A Type Of Surgery

So you have decided that you will be one of the 45,000 people who undergo weight loss surgery every year. But what type of surgery is for you? In order to determine what kind of surgery you want, you need to ask yourself many questions. What kind of eater are you and how overweight are you? Do you normally eat a lot of food or are you a sweet-eater? Do you eat healthy food, but just in large quantities? Do you need help cutting fats and sweets from your diet? Depending on what your eating habits are will determine what surgery is appropriate for you.

There are two types of weight loss surgeries: restrictive surgeries and a combination of restrictive and malabsorptive. Restrictive surgeries limit the amount of food that you can eat, but what you do eat is completely absorbed by your body. An example of a restrictive surgery is a Vertical Banded Gastroplasty (VBG).

A combination surgery of both restrictive and malabsorptive would be the Roux en-Y (RNY) gastric bypass surgery. The RNY is restrictive like the VBG but, in addition, it is also a malabsorptive procedure. The RNY limits the amount of food you can eat and, depending upon the amount of intestines bypassed, it will allow more food to pass out of the body with a smaller amount of calories, nutrients, and fat to be absorbed. Prior to my own surgery, I did a tremendous amount of research on the different surgery types and found the RNY to be far superior to the others for safe and permanent weight loss. The RNY is the most common weight loss surgery and is considered the "gold standard" of weight loss surgeries.

Each type of weight loss surgery has its advantages and disadvantages and each surgery is explained in depth in Chapters 10 thru 12.

Some are definitely better than others, and it is up to you to decide what is the best surgery for you. After you have made that decision, you may then be faced with the decision on whether the surgery is to be performed as an open procedure or laparoscopically. If you choose the laparoscopic surgery, your next challenge is to locate a surgeon in your area, or in an area to which you will be willing to travel, who performs laparoscopic surgery.

How Much Weight Can I Expect To Lose?

Weight loss will vary depending upon many factors. Studies have shown that RNY and duodenal switch patients lose the most weight. VBG patients lose less weight and lap band patients tend to average the least weight loss. Those who are heavier will lose weight more rapidly than those who are lighter. Men lose more weight than women. And younger patients lose faster than older patients. With an RNY, you can expect to lose approximately 80 percent of your excess weight and keep that weight off. Speaking very generally, you can expect to lose 15 to 20 pounds a month in the first few months and then your weight loss will begin to slow. The final 10 to 15 pounds are the hardest to lose. Often, these pounds are not lost without having plastic surgery done to remove excess skin.

> *RNY patients can expect to lose 80 percent of their excess weight; far more than through dieting.*

Although you can expect to lose 80 percent of your excess weight, surgeons consider you to be successful when you lose only 50 percent. In my own case, I have lost 100 percent of my excess weight and there are thousands of people who have done the same.

10
Roux en-Y (RNY) Gastric Bypass Surgery

The Roux en-Y (RNY) gastric bypass surgery is considered to be the "gold standard" in gastric bypass surgeries. It was named after a 19th century Swiss surgeon, Dr. Cesar Roux and was developed by Dr. Ward Griffin of the University of Kentucky in 1977. This type of surgery has the best success rate for weight loss, short-term as well as long-term, and has been endorsed by the National Institutes of Health. Further, the American Heart Association issued a paper in 1997 stating that in patients with a BMI greater than 40, surgery is the

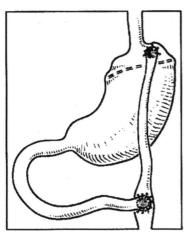

treatment of choice and the RNY surgery is the superior surgery. Although it is complex and difficult, it has the same mortality rate as any general surgery. This type of surgery produces a feeling of being full when eating a very small amount of food and produces a feeling of being satisfied. In many patients, a symptom called dumping, which is discussed later, results in an inability to eat excess sweets, which aids in the weight loss and weight maintenance process. Finally, the bypassing of part of the small intestines results in fewer calories being absorbed. The RNY surgery can be done as an open method (full incision) or laparoscopically. Although these methods are very different, the actual internal surgical procedure is the same. I will cover each method later in this chapter.

In the RNY procedure, the stomach is separated into two sections.

The upper part is made into a very small pouch that holds one to two ounces initially. It is about the size of a thumb. A normal stomach holds 40 to 50 ounces and is roughly the size of a human head. The new small pouch is positioned at the bottom of the esophagus and is very resistant to stretching. While the lower part of the stomach remains, nothing enters it. This lower part still produces gastric juices that eventually meet with the food and aid digestion. These two parts of the stomach are transected or completely separated. Each of the cut edges is closed by a method of stapling and sewing to eliminate the chance of leaks. A leak can be a very serious condition allowing food to enter the abdominal cavity causing severe infection. Scar tissue eventually forms at the stapled and sewn areas so that the upper pouch and lower stomach are permanently separated and sealed.

The staples that are used to close off the pouch and the stomach are made of titanium, which does not rust or corrode. The question often arises if these staples will interfere with or prevent an MRI at a later time. Because the staples are made from titanium, they do not have any effect on an MRI.

In the RNY, the old stomach still continues to produce gastric juices, even though no food enters it.

The small bowel is then cut about 18 inches below the old stomach. The end of the bowel that is not connected to the stomach is moved up and attached to the newly made pouch. After a hole is made in the stretched and moved bowel, the 18-inch bowel length that is connected to the lower stomach is attached to the part of the bowel now going to the new pouch, making a "Y" connection. This causes the duodenum and some of the jejunum sections of the intestines to be bypassed.

Although the old larger stomach does not receive any food, it does not wither and die. It still produces digestive fluids that eventually meet up with the food that is passed down from the new little pouch.

Instead of having the food be partially digested before moving into the intestines, this "Y" connection allows undigested food to be introduced directly into the lower part of the small intestines and mixed with gastric juices.

The opening between the new pouch and the intestines is called a stoma (or anastomosis). The surgeon creates this opening so that it is roughly the size of a pencil eraser or about 1/4 inch in diameter. This small outlet delays the emptying of food from the pouch and causes a feeling of fullness. Because the pyloric valve between the stomach and the duodenum is bypassed, it is important that the size of the stoma is small so that food will remain longer in the pouch. It is very important to chew food well so that it does not get caught in the stoma. If that happens, the stuck food will cause severe stomach cramps and vomiting. The food will almost always pass through by itself, but severe cases may require your surgeon to assist. If the stoma opening is found to be too small or closes because of swelling or a build up of scar tissue, an endoscopic procedure must be done to enlarge it.

Advantages of RNY Surgery

The main advantage of this surgery is its success rate. It is the most effective method of weight loss surgery and is approved by the National Institutes of Health. The short-term success rate with this surgery is 80 to 100 percent and the long-term success rate is almost as impressive. Success rate is defined as losing at least 50 percent of your excess weight. The ability to eat large amounts of food is lost forever. The physical limitation of the small pouch will cause you to vomit if you eat too much. During the early months after surgery, most people can only eat tiny amounts of food. This is mainly a result of the healing process of the stomach and intestines and helps to produce the "window of opportunity" when the most weight is lost. After this healing process is complete, you will find that you will gradually be able to eat more food at one sitting, but never like before the surgery. In most cases, this gradual ability to eat more will correspond to your body's desire to maintain your ideal weight.

A wonderful effect of this "window of opportunity" is that even though a person is only able to physically eat a small amount of food, the brain does not perceive a feeling of hunger. Because the food that is eaten quickly comes in contact with the lining of the upper small intestines, some surgeons believe that this causes the release of hormones, causing the patient to feel satisfied and no longer hungry. Ordinarily, this would not happen for 30 to 60 minutes but because it happens so rapidly with RNY patients, they avoid overeating. I found that I could go many hours without eating and not feel hungry. It is important to not force yourself to eat. As long as you are taking your vitamin supplements and drinking water, the small amounts of food you do eat will amply sustain you. Toward the end of your window of opportunity, you will find that a mild form of hunger will return, but not the ravenous hunger you may have experienced in the past.

Disadvantages of RNY Surgery

Disadvantages include the dumping syndrome that some people experience. This usually occurs when something sweet is eaten. In a normal stomach, the sweet food is partially digested from gastric juices. After surgery, sweet food enters the small intestines in a pure form and can cause symptoms of cramping, sweating, nausea, or vomiting. Dumping is sometimes viewed as an advantage, however, because it discourages people from eating sweets.

Other disadvantages include nutritional deficiencies, which can occur because part of the small intestines is bypassed and not all food is absorbed. A regimen of vitamins must be followed to avoid this. The stoma, or opening between the stomach and intestines can sometimes be too small, causing vomiting. In the early days after surgery, there is a small possibility of a leak occurring in the new small pouch or at the "Y" connection in the intestines. This is usually very evident immediately following surgery and is very serious, but can be repaired fairly easily if the leak does not heal on its own.

Laparoscopic Surgery

Laparoscopic surgery is sometimes referred to as minimally invasive surgery, less invasive surgery, or just lap surgery.

The goals of laparoscopic surgery are less pain, faster healing, less chance of infection, and faster recovery.

To perform laparoscopic (lap) surgery, a surgeon inserts a thin tubular telescope and a tiny high-resolution video camera into the abdomen through very small incisions. Four or five additional very small incisions are made in the abdomen and ports are inserted into these incisions so that the surgeon can do the actual surgery using long slender instruments. At the completion of the surgery, these small incisions are closed with stitches on the inside that dissolve in four to six weeks.

The tiny video camera at the end of one of the wands allows the surgeon to see inside the abdomen by magnifying and projecting the image onto a TV screen. The abdomen is first filled with gas so that the surgeon has room to work. Drs. Alan Wittgrove and Wesley Clark at the Alvarado Center for Surgical Weight Control in San Diego, California first used the laparoscopic procedure for gastric bypass surgery in 1993.

Laparoscopic surgery usually takes approximately 90 to 120 minutes as opposed to 60 to 90 minutes for the open procedure, which I will discuss next. Recovery time following laparoscopic surgery is usually less than for the open procedure. The hospital stay tends to be one to two days shorter, and many patients can return to work in about two to three weeks. A laparoscopic procedure does not reduce any of the risks of bariatric surgery, but it can reduce pain, recovery time, and scarring.

The laparoscopic technique cannot usually be performed on those patients who are over 400 pounds because of the difficulty of going through too much tissue during surgery. Additionally, the laparoscopic procedure cannot be done if the patient has excessive amounts of scarring or adhesions present from any previous abdominal surgeries. If this is the case, the surgeon may have to convert to an open procedure. A surgeon may also begin a laparoscopic procedure and then convert to an open procedure if enlarged organs prevent clear vision or if there is persistent bleeding.

Open Surgery

In the open procedure, an incision is made vertically from the breastbone to the navel, approximately 10 to 12 inches long. The surgeon's work is easier because all of the organs are in full view and the surgeon is able to work with less instrumentation.

While the open procedure is easier for the surgeon, it creates additional problems for the patient. The massive incision requires additional time in the hospital for recovery and additional time before a patient can return to work. Women seem to tolerate an open procedure better than men. Because of a difference in the center of gravity, men tend to carry their weight more in their abdomen, which puts more stress on the incision. Wearing a binder around the abdomen often helps with the stress on the incision; however some patients find binders too uncomfortable to wear.

The Lap vs. Open Debate

The surgery is the same whether it is done laparoscopically or as an open procedure. The debate merely centers on how the surgeon gains access to the stomach and intestines.

Those patients who have laparoscopic surgery feel it is better because it is less invasive. You are dealing with five or six tiny incisions rather than one large incision. The healing time is much faster with the lap and the post-operative pain is less. The hospital stay is usually one to two days less, and patients can go back to work or resume normal activities sooner.

There is also much less chance of infection with the lap. Laparoscopic procedures do not have the large open incision that is susceptible to complications. Many open patients have had their incision reopen, creating a source of wound infection. Also, when an incision reopens, it cannot be re-stitched. It must heal from the inside out, which is a very long process. These incision complications do not happen with a lap procedure. Should you have an open procedure and the incision opens, it is advisable to deal with a nurse who specializes in wound care. That expertise is invaluable. One additional complication with the open procedure is the increased risk of hernias.

A laparoscopic procedure reduces the risk of cardiopulmonary complications following gastric bypass surgery. Although complications in this area are rare, when they do occur, they are catastrophic.

Those who have open surgeries feel it is better because the surgeon can clearly see if there is anything wrong with the organs involved in the digestive process. The surgeon can see, touch and feel the patient's organs to determine if they are functioning correctly. Also, open procedures are less expensive than laparoscopic ones. The equipment and staff training involved cause the overall cost of a laparoscopic procedure to be at least $5,000 more than an open procedure.

An open procedure allows direct viewing of the internal organs.

Proximal, Medial and Distal

Proximal, medial, and distal refer to the amount of intestines that are bypassed. A proximal gastric bypass is the surgery that is normally performed. In this procedure, approximately 18 inches of intestines are bypassed. In a medial bypass, additional lengths of intestines are bypassed.

In distal bypass surgery, even more of the intestines are bypassed which results in less absorption. Although there is slightly better success with weight loss, there are complications that make the distal procedure somewhat less attractive. Malabsorption is increased which affects the amount of calcium and fat-soluble vitamins that are absorbed. This increases the risk of deficiencies and requires that patients be especially diligent about taking supplements.

Distal surgery patients often have bowel problems following surgery. Patients have more frequent bowel movements and sometimes have a distressing problem of passing very foul smelling gas. Two possible remedies include taking a very low dose of the antibiotic Flagyl or taking the medication Cipro, Simethicone, or Doxecycline. It may also help to decrease your intake of carbohydrates and fats and to eliminate sugar. This is because carbohydrates and sugars ferment in the intestines. Another remedy for gas is Chlorofresh, which is available in health stores. Yogurt may also help, because the yogurt culture may improve the flora in the stomach. Also Gas-X, acidophilus pills and Lactaid might help.

Although the length of the intestines bypassed is important for the patient to know about, the surgeon generally makes an educated decision on which to use based upon your weight and physiology. Although this will be his or her decision, you should discuss this with your surgeon so that you will have a more complete picture of what will be done to your body.

Fobi Pouch

The Fobi pouch is a modified open gastric bypass procedure developed by Dr. Mathias Fobi. He performs this procedure at the Center for the Surgical Treatment of Obesity in Hawaiian Gardens,

California. He also teaches this procedure to surgeons from across the country at this facility. The Fobi pouch is very similar to the RNY with a few exceptions. The Fobi pouch is a completely separated, or transected, pouch of less than 30 cc capacity. This is the same as the RNY. Where the Fobi pouch differs is in the stoma, or the opening to the intestines. The Fobi pouch uses a silastic ring to reinforce the stoma so that it does not stretch. In the Fobi pouch procedure, there is also a tube into the old stomach that is left in for 7 to 10 days. It is used for diagnostic purposes and to aid in relieving any complications. There is also somewhat more of the small intestines bypassed than in the normal RNY.

11
Lap Band: Laparoscopic Adjustable Silicone Gastric Banding

The lap band (or LASGB) is becoming the second most common form of weight loss surgery. It has been used in Europe for several years and had been in FDA trials at centers throughout the United States since 1995. It was expected to be approved by the FDA in the summer of 2000, however, the FDA required an additional year of testing. On Tuesday June 8th, 2001 the FDA approved the use of the lap band, but required that surgeons who insert the band must go through specialized training. The lap band is now available at practices throughout the United States.

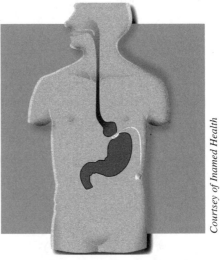

Courtesy of Inamed Health

In the lap band procedure, a silicone band is placed around the top of the stomach squeezing the stomach to make a small pouch. There is a narrow opening that allows food to slowly move from the upper small pouch to the lower stomach. Because the opening is narrow, food remains in the upper pouch providing the patient with a sensation of being full and satisfied.

When the lap band is inserted, there is a port that is also inserted just under the skin of the abdomen. This port connects to the lap band by tubing. The band itself has an inner lining that is filled with a saline solution. Through the port, the surgeon can inject more saline, which makes the band tighter if the patient wants to eat less or the surgeon can remove some of the saline if the patient wants to eat more

As with any procedures there are advantages and disadvantages. The following are some to consider:

Advantages

1. The surgery is less invasive. The gastrointestinal tract is not altered; therefore it is a safer procedure.
2. The hospital stay is shorter, usually 1 to 2 days, and patients can return to work in a week or two
3. Surgeons like the procedure because it is technically easier to perform and takes less time to perform.
4. Because the band is adjustable, the pouch can be customized so that the patient can eat as little or as much as desired.
5. If the patient is unhappy with the procedure, the band can be removed and the stomach generally returns to its original size and shape.
6. A patient wishing for no one to know he or she had weight loss surgery, can take off a week or two, return to work and appear that they are losing weight naturally, thereby ensuring their privacy.

Disadvantages

1. Patients lose less weight. In the clinical trials, the average loss of excess weight was 36-38% which is about half of what is generally lost with the RNY. However, as surgeons become more skilled and aftercare programs become more sophisticated, the weight loss should increase.
2. It is possible for the band to slip which results in the patient being able to eat more and regain weight, or the band slips and the pouch becomes so small that the patient cannot keep either food or liquid down.

3. It is easier for the patient to sabotage the procedure by drinking very high calorie liquids.
4. It is fairly easy for a patient to try to adjust the size of the pouch themselves. After they have seen it done once, it is fairly easy to do technically. This has had adverse results for some patients.
5. If the patient does want a revision to an RNY, there is a possibility that it could not be done laparoscopically because of a possible build up of scar tissue from the lap band.
6. Because the procedure is new, some insurance companies consider it experimental and use that as a justification to deny the claim.

In the June 2001 issue of the <u>Annals of Surgery</u>, a report was published on the lap band written by Eric J. DeMaria, MD; Harvey J. Sugerman, MD, et al, entitled "High Failure Rate After Laparoscopic Adjustable Silicone Gastric Banding for Treatment of Morbid Obesity", Vol. 233, p 809-818.

In the article the surgeons reported on 36 of their patients who have had lap bands placed from March 1996 to May 1998. The patients have been followed for up to 4 years. Of the 36 patients:

4   Had the lap band removed with no further treatment
11   Had the lap band removed and had the gastric bypass done
8   Want the lap band removed and want the gastric bypass because of inadequate weight loss.
6   Are still morbidly obese after 2 years but do not want any further surgery.
4   Have achieved a BMI of less than 35 or at least a 50% reduction in excess weight. This is an 11% success rate.

The remaining patients have been lost after 2 years to follow up, but at last report had maintained only an 18% weight loss.

A later study was reported by Dr. Richard Rubenstein of the State University of New York at Stony Brook. In this study, published in the journal, "Obesity Surgery," June 2002 issue, Dr. Rubenstein reports more favorable results than those of Dr. DeMaria.

His study involved 63 patients who underwent banding between March 1999 and June 2001. Of the 63 patients, 18 had complications, which were relatively minor (1 gastric perforation which was resolved, 5 port problems, 9 band slippage, and 3 infections). What was especially interesting was the way people lost weight. With RNY gastric bypass surgery, patients lose their greatest amount of weight during the first 12 to 18 months, stop losing and then tend to regain 10 or 15 pounds over the next 3 years until they stabilize.

With the lap band, the weight loss was gradual over the 3-year study. Patients averaged 27.2% loss of their excess weight at 6 months, 38.3% at 1 year, 46.4% at 2 years and 53.6% at 3 years. Dr. Rubenstein concluded that his practice had achieved results comparable to those in Europe, and that optimal results were achieved with careful patient selection, a refined surgical technique, and a long-term patient management program.

Now that the lap band is becoming more widely available and surgeons are becoming more adept at the surgical technique, the lap band will be one more option for patients to consider in their choice of surgeries. And there are some patients who have been pleased with their results.

To learn more about the lap band, visit the Inamed website **http://www.inamed.com/products/obesity/us/patient/patient.html.** Inamed is a manufacturer of the lap band.

12

Other Less Common Surgeries and Procedures

Biliopancreatic Diversion with Duodenal Switch

Biliopancreatic Diversion with Duodenal Switch (BPD/DS) uses both restriction and malabsorption to accomplish weight loss. In this surgery, approximately 2/3rds of the stomach is removed so that it holds approximately four to six ounces. The stomach is separated along what is referred to as the greater curvature resulting in a long incision line. Because the stomach is reduced so drastically, patients do not feel as much hunger as they experienced before. The 1/3rd of the stomach

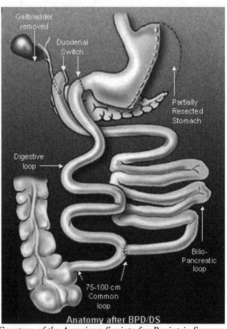

Courtsey of the American Society for Bariatric Surgery

remaining continues to function just as it did prior to surgery.

Food enters the reduced stomach and continues into the small intestines by going through the pyloric valve. The pyloric valve regulates the emptying of the contents of the stomach into the intestines. Because the pyloric valve remains, patients do not experience the dumping syndrome that is troublesome to many RNY patients. The intestines are rearranged so that one portion of the intestines carries the food and the other portion of the intestines carries the bile and pancreatic juices. These digestive juices meet up with the food in a short common channel just before entering the large intestines. It is in this short common channel that absorption takes place. Therefore fewer calories are absorbed, especially calories from fat. More absorption of calcium, iron and B-12 occurs because a portion of the duodenum remains in the digestive tract.

Of all the weight loss surgeries, the BPD/DS has the greatest opportunity for weight loss.

Advantages
1. Patients can eat much more normally, consuming larger amounts of food.
2. Because the pyloric valve remains, the dumping syndrome is not an issue.
3. Because the top part of the stomach and intestines are left intact, it is not necessary to create an anastomosis (stoma) between the pouch and the intestines. Therefore the problem of the stoma becoming smaller from scar tissue or clogging from eating something difficult to digest is not an issue.
4. Patients have the greatest amount of weight loss, averaging over 80% of excess weight.

Disadvantages
1. Because the incision line of the stomach is much longer in the BPD/DS, there is a much greater chance of leakage from the operation, which is a potentially dangerous condition.
2. The surgery employs far more malabsorption than the RNY, therefore nutritional issues are more critical, especially in the absorption of protein.
3. Patients are more prone to diarrhea and foul smelling gas. This does however tend to correct itself over time.
4. The stomach portion of the surgery is not reversible because the actual stomach is removed.
5. Because the BPD/DS has not as yet been endorsed by the

National Institutes of Health, obtaining insurance coverage can be more difficult.

Vertical Banded Gastroplasty

While the frequency of RNY Surgery far exceeds all other types of weight loss surgeries, some surgeons still prefer the Vertical Banded Gastroplasty (VBG). Dr. Edward Mason developed the VBG when he tried to find a safe yet effective method of weight loss surgery. Dr. Mason is known as the father of weight loss surgery. The VBG is a variation of the former stomach stapling method.

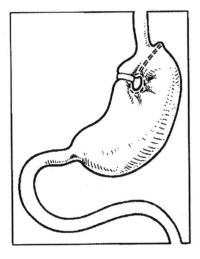

Dr. Mason developed the Vertical Banded Gastroplasty when he realized that the stomach wall, with the lesser curvature, was thicker and less likely to stretch. Therefore making the pouch out of this part of the stomach decreased the possibility of the pouch becoming larger. To make the pouch, he stapled the pouch vertically rather than horizontally, then placed a band horizontally at the bottom of this pouch to make an opening to the lower stomach.

It is widely recognized that the Vertical Banded Gastroplasty is not as effective as the Roux en-Y gastric bypass, but some surgeons, and patients alike, prefer it because they believe it is technically easier to perform. There is no cutting and moving of the intestines. It is a purely restrictive procedure with no malabsorption because none of the intestines are bypassed. People who have the VBG do not experience dumping syndrome and therefore, are not bothered by sweet foods or sugar. This of course can be viewed as both an advantage and a disadvantage! Dumping is not a pleasant experience, however it does act as a deterrent to eating foods high in sugar. The Vertical Banded Gastroplasty has been approved by the National Institutes of Health.

About 30 percent of patients undergoing Vertical Banded Gastroplasty achieve normal weight, and about 80 percent achieve some degree of weight loss. However, because the procedure does not create the sense of satisfaction that patients having the RNY experience, some patients are not able to change their eating habits and are unable to lose the weight that they had hoped. Reports indicate a 43 to 48 percent loss of excess weight for the VBG as opposed to a 66 to 80 percent loss for the RNY gastric bypass surgery. Also, according to a study done by the Mayo Clinic, only 38 percent of patients were able to maintain their weight loss of 50 percent or more, 3 years after their surgery.

Disadvantages to this surgery include the possibility of excessive vomiting which is reported in up to 50 percent of patients. Patients need to chew food very carefully. Because of the anatomy of the VBG, patients seem to be predisposed to gastroesophageal reflux disease. Also, the band may slip, erode or break and the staple line can break down, causing weight to be regained. Another disadvantage is the ability to easily sabotage the effectiveness of the surgery by drinking very high calorie drinks such as regular soda or milk shakes because they comfortably slide down and do not cause vomiting.

Mini Gastric Bypass (Also Known as Billroth II)

The mini gastric bypass was performed years ago, but has been discontinued by most surgeons as being unsafe. The surgery connects a small vertical, divided pouch to a loop of proximal small bowel. Dr. Edward Mason, University of Iowa College of Medicine, warns that this results in bile and pancreatic juices refluxing into the stomach pouch. Similar concerns have been expressed by Drs. Mervyn Deitel and Henry Buchwald, both past presidents of the American Society for Bariatric Surgery; as well as Dr. James K. Champion, Mercer University School of Medicine; Dr. Barry Fisher, University of

Nevada School of Medicine; Dr. Harvey Sugerman, Medical College of Virginia; Dr. Fafael Capella, University of Medicine and Dentistry of New Jersey; and Dr. Patricia Choban, Ohio State University Medical Center. Dr. Champion states that the loop bypass channels bile and digestive juice into the esophagus where it can cause reflux esophagitis, ulceration, and esophageal cancer over a period of years. Many who have had this surgery have required extensive revisions to correct the severe problems that they are experiencing.

Revisions

A revision is a surgical procedure that changes you from one type of surgery to another. The most common revision is from the Vertical Banded Gastroplasty to the Roux en-Y. Some VBG patients, about 28 percent according to Dr. Mathias Fobi, experience problems with the banding slipping or breaking causing weight gain or they experience excessive vomiting. They therefore have a revision performed.

Most insurance companies have the same requirement for revision surgery as they do for the original surgery. You must be 100 pounds overweight or have a BMI of 40 or above. However, whatever the reason, revision surgery is not optimum. It is far better to select the best type of surgery for you initially, so that you are not faced with the ordeal of a revision.

Reversals

A reversal involves undoing the original surgery. A VBG is easier to reverse than an RNY because in the VBG, no rerouting of the intestinal tract has been done. It is extremely rare, but there have been patients who have had their RNY's undone. These are usually people who could not deal with the psychological changes involved with such a permanent change in eating. After a reversal, it is not likely that the intestinal tract will function the way it did prior to the surgery. Again, it is important to make sure that weight loss surgery is what you want.

13
Locating A Surgeon and Preparing For Your First Visit

What can be more important than the surgeon who performs your surgery? You are at the mercy of your surgeon's training, intelligence, skill, focus, and concentration. As weight loss surgery becomes more popular, bariatric centers and hospital departments are proliferating as the medical community jumps on the bandwagon. We all want the very best, but how do we know who is the best. Unfortunately, not every surgeon can be the best. You want to ensure that the surgeon you select is board-certified and experienced in this type of surgery. It is a risky venture to be the first patient on which your surgeon is performing this operation. You want a surgeon who specializes in bariatric surgery, not one who does this occasionally along with other surgical procedures. You also want a surgeon who will provide you with a full range of services including long term follow-up, support group services, nutritional therapy, and referrals for psychological counseling. This will provide you with your greatest chance of success.

Referral From A Friend

One of the best ways to locate a surgeon is to seek out friends or acquaintances that have had weight loss surgery in the last few years. Surgeons who are recommended by their patients will generally have a good reputation. This makes the entire process much easier, because in a sense you know what you are getting. A person who had a bad experience is not likely to give a glowing recommendation. When you consider the seriousness of weight loss surgery, it is very comforting to actually know a person that has succeeded in losing weight because of the work that this surgeon has done.

Primary Care Physician Referral

Some people select a surgeon because of a referral from their primary care physician. However, what if your primary care physician is less than enthusiastic about your decision? Also, some primary care physicians are not very knowledgeable about the latest advances in weight loss surgery; therefore you may be offered little help there.

So where do you go to find an excellent local surgeon who performs the type of weight loss surgery in which you are interested? I have included some excellent resources to help you in your search. Don't find just one and then stop. Your body and your life are at stake here, so do some diligent research with several surgeons and then select the best one for you.

Association for Morbid Obesity Support

This web site, **http://www.obesityhelp.com/morbidobesity** that has over 120,000 members, is an excellent source for information regarding surgeons. Not only does the site list surgeons by state and city, it also lists the insurance plans that they accept as well as comments from patients. These patients have included their personal stories, so you can read about any complications that they may have had. Patients also include their email address so you can communicate with them regarding questions you may have.

OSSG

The Obesity Surgery Support Group (OSSG) is an online discussion group that deals with all aspects of weight loss surgery and is subscribed to by more than 5,000 members. Any question can be thrown out to the group for specific information or opinion. A simple question stating where you are from and asking for the name of a good local weight loss surgeon can yield important and useful information.

To join OSSG, go to **http://groups.yahoo.com/group/ossg.**

The American Society for Bariatric Surgery

The American Society for Bariatric Surgery **http://www.asbs.org** is a professional organization for surgeons performing bariatric surgery. To be a member of this organization, a surgeon needs only to pay dues, so membership does not necessarily ensure competence. However, membership does indicate a level of involvement and commitment to professional standards. This website will supply you with names of bariatric surgeons by city and state which will give you an additional place to start.

Your Insurance Company

Although your insurance company will not recommend a surgeon, they may tell you what surgeons in your network specialize in bariatric surgery. They may also tell you that weight loss surgery is not a covered benefit. Do not necessarily believe them at this point. You have a long way to go before you burn that bridge.

Surgeon Seminar

With weight loss surgery becoming so popular, many surgeons now require that you attend an informational seminar prior to having an appointment. This is an excellent way to get an idea about how knowledgeable the surgeon is, what rapport you may have, and how he or she responds to questions. Another option is to attend the support group sponsored by your surgeon. These are usually open to those who are just considering surgery. Here you will have an opportunity to meet patients who have gone through the surgery. Do not be shy about asking these patients any questions you may have. I have found that since most patients are so excited about their weight loss, they are willing to talk to anyone about their life changing achievement. Also ask for phone numbers and email addresses so that you can follow up with additional questions.

Your First Visit With the Surgeon

I was very nervous the day I first met with Dr. Schauer. I was concerned that I might not weigh enough, or have enough co-morbidities and that he would not accept me as a patient. Others have shared with me that they felt just the opposite. They were concerned that they might weigh too much and have so many co-morbidities that they also might not be accepted for surgery. But Dr. Schauer was wonderful. He put me at ease immediately, answered all of my questions and offered the opinion that I was an excellent candidate who should fully expect to reach goal weight.

I had done a tremendous amount of research and arrived at my appointment prepared with about 30 written questions that would give me details about Dr. Schauer's particular technique. It is essential that you also be prepared for your interview by writing out your questions before you arrive. When the surgeon walks in, you will probably be very nervous. After all, this person could be giving you a new lease on life and be fulfilling your lifelong dreams of being thin. If you try to remember all your questions, all of the information can confuse or frighten you and those questions can go right out of your head. If you remember an important question when you are halfway home, it may be difficult to get in touch with the surgeon. Write your questions down beforehand. Start a folder of all of your weight loss surgery research and information and jot your questions in this folder.

My husband attended that first appointment with me. Prior to that appointment, he was anxious for me and had many of his own questions. After meeting with Dr. Schauer and hearing his answers, he was relieved and very enthusiastic about the surgery. It was a major turning point for him. Even if your spouse is comfortable with the surgery, having your spouse, a family member or friend with you during this first meeting is a great idea. You will have a backup to clarify your understanding of what was discussed. It will also help to clear up any misconceptions that either of you may have.

Be prepared for your first visit with your surgeon by reading this book thoroughly and having your own list of written questions.

14
To Tell or Not to Tell

This is a very difficult and personal decision to make. Who do you tell about your surgery and when do you tell them?

Your Family

You will of course tell your spouse or significant other of your decision to have weight loss surgery, as well as your children. The approval of our immediate family is very important to us. Also, these are the people whom we will rely on to care for us immediately after our surgery. Because these people care for us and love us, they will tend to be very concerned. They probably have no knowledge of weight loss surgery, or worse, they know of the dangerous procedures done during the early years of weight loss surgery and think that this is the procedure that you are going to have performed. Remember your reactions when you first heard about this surgery and how much you had to learn to understand it. Give your family that chance to learn so that it will be easier for them to accept your decision. They may not be able to understand that for someone who is severely overweight, losing that weight is a lot more involved than to just stop eating. Tell them that the National Institutes of Health recommends weight loss surgery as the only effective means of weight control for those who are morbidly obese. Talk to them about health issues and how this surgery is a chance for you to live a longer, healthier life. Give them a copy of this book and have them read Chapter 34, To All "Significant Others." If there is a local support group, have your family members attend so that they can talk to some of the patients who have been through the surgery. Have them go with you to meet with your surgeon so that they have an opportunity to ask questions and express concerns. If, however, despite all of your efforts, your family remains opposed, then you will need to decide what is in your own best interest, and act accordingly.

Initially, my husband was very opposed to my surgery. But he went to every appointment I had with the surgeon and to all of the support group meetings as well. The more that he was involved, the more that he understood. This helped to ease his mind so that he could be there for me and be tremendously supportive. Not all spouses are that supportive. They are dealing with their fears that you will die or that you, as well as your life together, will change. My husband understood that this was my life and my body and ultimately I was the one to decide what was in my best interest. What he wanted most for me was to be healthy and happy.

Extended family can be more of a problem. Family dynamics will sometimes play a role here, which has nothing to do with your surgery. Sisters may not want you to relinquish your position of the "poor fat" sister. Aunts, uncles, or cousins who are unfamiliar with your struggles to lose weight may not be sympathetic. Your role will be changing and your family may have a difficult time adjusting to it. Deal as best as you can. Family issues are difficult. If they are more than you are able to cope with, seek counseling to assist you.

Your Friends

Your true friends will be there for you because they want the best for you. But many of your friends are used to dealing with you in ways that involve huge amounts of food. You may have a routine of going out to eat or sitting together over a pan of brownies and devouring the whole thing. Many of these behaviors will be changing. As you lose weight, you will want to become more active and your friends may not be able to or want to join you. Also, as you lose weight, your personality may change as you find more self-confidence. Many friendships cannot survive all of these changes.

By doing your own research, you can separate fact from fiction when you hear horror stories.

Be prepared to hear many horror stories as your friends try to talk you out of your decision to have surgery. Everyone seems to know someone who had this surgery who died or had horrible complications. Or they may know someone who had "stomach stapling" done years ago and they regained all of their weight. Stomach stapling has become something of an urban legend. It seems that everyone has heard the term, "stomach stapling," and always associates it with the previous horrors or failures of weight loss surgeries performed years ago. Remember that weight loss surgery has changed greatly over the years and the RNY gastric bypass surgery is a permanent, successful, and modern procedure.

Your Colleagues

I chose not to tell any of my colleagues what surgery I was having. This was for a number of reasons. First of all, I did not want to deal with any negativity. I did not want to hear any old horror stories, especially since I had done my own research on modern procedures and had talked to current patients.

I also did not want anyone to believe that I was taking off six weeks from work for what he or she might believe was cosmetic surgery to feed my own vanity. Not many of my colleagues understood the severity of my back pain and that if I did not do something about it soon, I might not be able to continue working. These were the people who would be holding up my end at work and I was concerned that they might be resentful. I chose to deal with it, if there was anything to deal with, when I returned from my medical leave. I should have known, however, that everyone in the end was extremely supportive. I am fortunate to work with some very special people.

Finally, I did not want to tell anyone because I feared that, despite all of my knowledge about my surgery and its success rate, I might be the one person in the world that would not lose weight. How could I deal with the embarrassment of another weight loss failure?

In the medical excuse for your employer, your surgeon does not have to specify what kind of surgery you are having.

The letter from my surgeon to my employer merely said that I was having surgery. Most people believed that I was having a hysterectomy. When I returned from my surgery and was rapidly losing weight, many people believed that I had cancer. But as they saw me get the spring back in my step, and then thrive into the picture of health, they knew that it wasn't cancer. When people would ask me how I lost all my weight, I always proudly told them that I had gastric bypass surgery. If they looked confused, I told them that it was weight loss surgery. I wanted to spread the word that this surgery provides hope for the morbidly obese where there was no hope.

15
Pre-Op Testing

Many surgeons require pre-op testing because, as a morbidly obese patient, your chances of complications during surgery are greatly increased. Some surgeons require more tests than others. Your surgeon, therefore, wants an accurate and detailed picture of your physical condition so that there will be few or no surprises during surgery. Often, people are concerned about these tests, thinking that they will "fail" a test and be ineligible for this surgery. This is extremely rare. You should be aware, however that some surgeons will only operate on patients who exhibit no unusual co-morbidities while others are confident enough to take on the more difficult cases.

Upper GI

The upper GI or barium swallow test examines the upper gastrointestinal tract and small bowel for any problems. In this test you are asked to drink a barium mixture that has a chalky taste. As you drink the liquid, the barium coats your gastrointestinal tract. Because x-rays do not pass through barium, when an x-ray picture is taken, your entire tract appears dark. A fluorescent screen converts the dark silhouette to a visible light. The radiologist, assisted by the technologist, can watch the path of the barium as it moves through your tract.

Sonogram

This test will check the condition of your gall bladder and whether it needs to be removed during surgery. Because of the frequent loss and regain of weight that we have all experienced as a result of yo-yo dieting, our gall bladders often contain gallstones and need to be removed. If needed, this can be done at the same time as the weight loss surgery. In this test, a technician moves a microphone-like device over the abdominal area. This device produces and receives high frequency sound waves, of such high frequency that we cannot hear them. The sound waves reflect off your organs and produce an image on a video screen that can be studied to determine any problems.

Cardio Exam

You will probably be referred to a cardiologist who will determine the condition of your heart. The test may be as simple as taking your family history along with an electrocardiogram and listening to your heart with a stethoscope, to a more extensive evaluation such as a stress test. If you have taken the diet drug Phen-Fen for more than three months in the past, you may also be required to have an echocardiogram to check for any heart valve damage.

Psychological Evaluation

You may be required to meet with a psychologist to determine if you are mentally and emotionally stable to have this surgery, and to evaluate your ability to adjust to the changes necessary after your surgery. Remember that it is very common for morbidly obese people to be depressed. You are probably dealing with tremendous feelings of failure, low self-esteem and often, chronic pain. Therefore, depression is common and not something that you need to feel will disqualify you from having surgery. Some people have unrealistic expectations of how their lives will change after having lost a tremendous amount of weight, and sometimes these issues will be dealt with during an evaluation. Becoming thin will not cure all of your problems. A typical psych evaluation involves a discussion session followed by a lengthy written test. The test is looking to see if you are either suicidal or psychotic, if you have a drug or alcohol abuse problem, or if you have an eating disorder. The session lasts about one hour. If you feel comfortable with the psychologist, you may want to make further appointments to deal with issues of eating, self-image and changing relationships. The psychologist is probably accustomed to dealing with these issues if he or she was recommended by your surgeon.

Chest X-Ray

A chest x-ray of your heart and lungs is done to help determine the health of these organs.

Dietician

Your surgeon may refer you to a nutritionist or dietician who will offer some guidance on post-operative eating. A good dietician, who is knowledgeable, understands the issues that weight loss surgery patients face, and how best to deal with eating post-operatively, can be a tremendous help. More bariatric practices are including a dietician on their team.

Endocrinologist

If you suffer from diabetes, you will be required to see an endocrinologist for an evaluation of your system.

Blood Tests

Blood work is usually required within 30 days of your surgery. The required tests will vary with different surgeons and with your own physical condition. Before any blood work is done, check with your physician or surgeon's office to find out if it is necessary to fast prior to the test. Blood will be drawn from a vein in your arm, usually a vial or two. Here are the tests that are often required of patients having weight loss surgery:
CBC (Complete Blood Cell Count) is the most common blood test.

This test counts the types of blood cells present in a volume of your blood. The test measures hemoglobin, white and red blood cells and platelets. This test can detect anemia, infections or leukemia.

Lipid Profile measures the amount of fat present in your blood. It measures cholesterol, HDL and triglycerides. This test could indicate a risk of coronary artery disease.

SMAC 24 is also known as a Comprehensive Metabolic Panel and is becoming more common. This test requires fasting for eight hours prior to the test. The test covers albumin, albumin/globulin ratio, alkaline phosphatase, and aspartate transaminase, bilirubin total, bun/creatinine ratio, calcium, carbon dioxide, chloride, creatinine, globulin, glucose potassium, protein total, sodium, and urea nitrogen (bun).

Blood Chemistry Group will analyze electrolytes and blood sugar. It will include a liver function test by checking bilirubin and a kidney function test to check levels of uric acid and creatinine. Usually levels of albumin are also checked.

Coagulation tests are done to determine the rate that your blood clots.

Oral Glucose Tolerance Test is required if you are diabetic or suspect that you may be diabetic. You are required to fast for at least eight hours prior to this test. The test is done in four segments in thirty-minute intervals and checks insulin levels, glucose and C-peptide.

Thyroid Studies measure the levels of thyroid stimulating hormones present in the blood.

Levels of calcium, magnesium and iron are also checked.

Sleep Apnea

It is very common for people who are morbidly obese to suffer from some degree of sleep apnea, a condition in which you stop breathing repeatedly during your sleep. When you stop breathing, your muscles jerk you out of a deep sleep enough so that you start to breathe again. As a result of this light and restless sleep, you are very tired the next day.

If you do not suspect that you have sleep apnea, you may just need an oximetric study done while you sleep at home. This single night test is done using a small machine about the size of a laptop computer. After you place a strip under your nose and attach a clip to your index finger, you go to sleep normally. This test checks the percentage of oxygen present in your blood stream during the night, while you sleep.

If your oxygen levels are found to be low on this test, you will be required have a more extensive sleep study called a polysomnography that is done while you sleep in a laboratory setting. Sensors are attached all over your body, including your head. You are then left to go to sleep and you are monitored via the sensors as well as filmed. A major complaint about this test is trying to wash the gel out of your hair! Some sleep labs use acetone or acetone-based fingernail polish remover to remove the gel and it will not hurt your hair.

The polysomnography test records the amount of time that you spend in stage 1 sleep, stage 2 sleep, stage 3/4 sleep and REM (rapid eye movement) sleep by monitoring your brain waves. The number of times that you awaken during the night, your respiration, muscle tension, and the amount of oxygen in your blood is recorded. An audio monitor records how much you snore or gasp. Sleep apnea is very serious. If you are found to have this condition, you will be fitted with a C-Pap (Continuous Positive Airway Pressure), which is a device that aids in your breathing. A C-Pap blows air into your nose via an air mask, keeping the airway open. A Bi-Pap (Bi-Level) is for more severe cases of sleep apnea. This device blows air at two different pressures. The inhale pressure is higher and the exhale pressure is lower.

The reason that sleep apnea is serious is that after surgery you will be taken off of a ventilator and you will have to breathe on your own.

If you have sleep apnea, your brain may forget to tell your lungs to breathe. During your recovery, your respiration will be closely monitored.

16
The Last Supper:
Will I Ever Be Able To Eat Again?

After all the research you have done, one fact stands out above all others. It has become very clear that your eating habits will drastically change after the surgery. You fear that your lifelong friend of food will be lost to you forever. Because of this natural emotional feeling, there is a great tendency to have a series of "last suppers" as you wait for your surgery date. Many fears of missing food forever flood your mind. You know about dumping so it is natural to want to eat all the sweets you can. The thoughts keep going through your mind that, after surgery, you won't be able to eat this, or you won't be able to eat that, so you consume everything in great quantities with the mistaken idea that this will be the last memory of food that must stay with you for the rest of your life. Unfortunately the only thing you gain is the added weight as you eat your way to the operating room.

Dealing with the emotional bond I had with food, was one of the hardest things for me to overcome prior to my surgery.

Food has no doubt been a big part of your life. You use food to celebrate. You use food when you are bored. You use food as a great comfort when you are sad. How will you deal with these emotions when you cannot use food in the way that you have in the past? You love food, so in the days and weeks leading up to surgery, you may find yourself eating more than ever. I know because that is exactly what I did. I knew at the time it was not a good idea, but I couldn't help myself. I was hysterical. I wanted the surgery so badly, yet I was fearful. How did I deal with these emotions? I ate everything in sight.

It really is to your advantage to be in the best shape possible when you have surgery. Weight loss surgery is a major undertaking and morbidly obese people are at a greater risk than those of normal weight, any time they are facing surgery. If you can lose some weight, it is definitely a positive. Some surgeons require all of their patients to lose 10 percent of their weight prior to surgery. One binge after another is not the way to go. If you can keep this tendency under control, you will be better off – and a better person than I was!

I have now discovered that I can eat almost anything, just in smaller quantities. So all of those "last suppers" to eat all of the foods that I thought I would never be able to eat again, were totally unnecessary.

17
Getting Ready For Your Hospital Discharge

Before you go to the hospital, have a few things on hand for when you get home. You don't want to go shopping the same day as you are discharged from the hospital. You also need to make some arrangements to ensure a smooth transition back to your everyday life.

Food Items

Have a couple of cans of chicken broth, a bottle of apple juice, sugar free Popsicles, some herbal tea (peppermint and chamomile), and some sugar free gelatin. That should do it. Don't over stock on things that you think you will like.

Be prepared, but don't overstock. Eleven months after my surgery, I finally used the last of my cans of broth.

Medicines

Have your prescriptions refilled for any medications that you normally take. Although losing weight will probably mean that you will soon be off of many of your medications, it is very important that you do not stop taking them until you have been instructed to do so by your physician. Some people have tried to stop their medications on their own and have gotten into serious health problems.

If your surgeon is prescribing any pain medication for your use at home, ask your surgeon if you can have the prescription early so that you can get it filled prior to going into the hospital. There is nothing worse than traveling home in pain and having to stop at a drug store to get a prescription filled. Also, the prescriptions may be for something that is not readily available. My surgeon prescribes Roxicet, a liquid form of Percocet which is not normally available. My pharmacist had to order it and it took a few days to arrive. If I were home from the hospital and had to wait a couple of days for pain medication, I would not have been a happy camper. You may also want to have some over-the-counter liquid pain reliever available. Ask your surgeon for a recommendation.

Arrangements For Your Children

If you have small children, try to make arrangements for babysitting for at least a week after you return home, unless your spouse is able to completely take over. You will not be able to lift the little ones to give them the care they need. You will need someone to care for you, rather than you caring for others. Some patients come home and are in great shape soon after they arrive, but this is not something you can count on. Even if you are feeling good, you should not lift anything over five pounds until your surgeon clears you.

Take Care Of Loose Ends

Pay all of the bills that you can prior to surgery so that you do not have to bother about it when you return home. Return any library books or video rentals. The idea is to get all the loose ends taken care of before the surgery so you can just rest afterward.

Furniture And Equipment

Consider investing in or renting a recliner. Some people are able to sleep in bed like normal, but if the pain is too uncomfortable and you cannot, a recliner is invaluable. Some people rent a hospital bed and in some situations your insurance may cover the cost. When you do return to sleeping in bed, using a body pillow will make you more comfortable.

Be sure you have an accurate thermometer at home. If you suspect a fever upon your return from the hospital, you will want to know for sure. A fever above 100 degrees is an indication that something serious may be wrong, so this elevated temperature must be reported immediately to your surgeon.

If your surgery is open, speak to your surgeon about using a stomach binder. These can provide much needed support during the first couple of weeks following surgery. Binders are available at many drug stores and medical supply stores.

A shower chair can be an important safety device for the first week following your surgery, especially if you will be showering at home alone. You will have gone through general anesthesia, which normally leaves you a little disoriented until all of the effects have worn off. This may take a week or two. You may also feel quite weak from having gone through major surgery and from now being on a 100 percent liquid diet.

Breathing Exercises

As soon as possible prior to your surgery, start doing deep breathing exercises as much and as often as you can. Take a deep breath and hold it for a count of ten and exhale slowly through pursed lips like you are blowing out a candle. You should also practice coughing which is something that you will be doing a lot of in the hospital. You have to cough as a part of your hospital breathing exercises. If your lungs are clear and well oxygenated going in to surgery, there is less chance of developing pneumonia or collapsed air-sacs in the lungs.

The first day after my surgery, I looked at the nurse and said, "Cough, what do you mean, cough? Don't you know I just had stomach surgery?"

Preparation If Facing Surgery Alone

If you are facing this surgery alone, without help from family or friends, there are special considerations for you to be aware of. First of all, have your home prepared for your return. Have your laundry done, your home clean, your bills paid, your liquids available and your prescriptions filled. Have your medications and vitamins available. Buy some magazines and some books for your recuperation. If you have a VCR, pre-tape a number of movies and programs so you will have ready access to entertainment. Do not borrow books from the library or rent movies. You may not feel up to returning them when they are due.

Be sure that your surgeon knows that you have no help at home and you want to stay in the hospital as long as you can. Do not be in a rush to get out of there. Depending upon your co-morbidities, you may want to speak to your surgeon about going into an extended care or rehabilitation facility for a few days after you are released from the hospital. Also, speak to your insurance company about arranging for some form of home care. If you are a member of a church, inquire if there is a group whose members might stop in to check on you.

If you live alone, consider going into a rehabilitation facility for a few days following your hospital discharge. You will be so much stronger and feel more confident when you do arrive home.

Finally, if your surgeon has a support group, ask if there is a committee of the support group that is available to offer help. These people are known as "Angels" and have volunteered to provide assistance to those who have just had surgery. You may be a very independent person, but now is not the time to exercise that independence. Seek out and accept help. If you do very well after surgery, you can send all your help home. But if you do worse than expected and have not made arrangements, you could be completely miserable.

18
Your Before Statistics

The day before your surgery, weigh yourself, take your measurements and take some "before" pictures. I cannot stress how important this is. A record of how far you have come can help you to deal with times of discouragement. I recommend that you use either a digital camera or have your regular camera film developed with a computer disk included. You may want to send email to someone to show your progress or you might want to display the photos on the Internet. Displaying your "before" pictures may seem to be the last thing you would ever want to do, but you will find that, as you show everyone how far you have come, you will feel proud.

As painful as it is, take plenty of "before" pictures. They will be your source of inspiration for years to come.

Weighing yourself is obvious. You will want to have a record of where you started from with your weight. However, as you are losing weight, it is sometimes hard to remember what your former self really looked like. You will feel like you don't really look that different. Well you do, and your pictures will show you that. Friends will say that they see a difference in your face. Well look at your before pictures and you will start to see it also. Take some shots from the front, side and back in a variety of outfits including the dreaded bathing suit. Take another set after six months and then after one year. These will become some of your most prized pictures.

Measurements are also important. Often the scale does not give you accurate information on your progress. You may reach a plateau during which you are not losing any weight, but you may be losing inches during that time. I was on a plateau for three weeks near the

88

beginning of my journey. Although I did not lose a pound during that period of time, my clothing size went down and I lost several inches. If you are taking regular measurements, for instance every two weeks, then the plateaus will be easier to deal with and you will be much less discouraged.

19
Your Wish List:
It's Time For Dreams To Come True

Before your surgery, make a list of all the things you would like to do after you have lost weight. Sometimes we think that weight loss surgery is only about losing weight, but it is so much more than just that. It is about having a vibrant and exciting new life. It is about doing the things that might have been impossible in the past. Here are some things that you could put on your list:

> ➤ Walk up the stairs without getting short of breath
> ➤ Play with your children
> ➤ Go to an amusement park and have the safety bar go down
> ➤ Ride in an airplane and not need a seat belt extension
> ➤ Cut down or eliminate your medications
> ➤ Paint your toenails
> ➤ Stop worrying that the chair that you are sitting in might fall apart beneath you
> ➤ Stop worrying that the restaurant that you are going to might have only booths
> ➤ Fit in a bathtub and have water on both sides
> ➤ Shop in a store for regular sized people
> ➤ Buy clothes because you like them not just because they are big enough
> ➤ Not be the biggest person in any room
> ➤ Cross your legs
> ➤ Ride a bicycle
> ➤ Skate
> ➤ Have so much energy you wake up feeling ready to rock and roll

During the times when you may get discouraged and feel that you are not making any real progress, take out your list and rejoice in how far you have come by checking off the items you can now accomplish. Look at each of the other items as a personal challenge to overcome. From my own experience and the experience of many of the people I have come in contact with, I know that you will prevail.

20
Surgery Considerations

What To Take To The Hospital

There are several things that you may want to take with you to the hospital to make your stay more comfortable.

> **A pillow** - You will probably rest more comfortably if you take your own pillow with you to the hospital. A pillow is also important to hold against your stomach when you have to cough, which is part of your breathing exercise. A large, soft teddy bear is also good for this. Riding home from the hospital can be much less traumatic if you hold a pillow, or a teddy bear, against your tummy. Some people prefer to use a neck pillow while in the hospital.

> **A fan** - Many people are troubled by heat in the hospital and appreciate having a small fan with them.

> **Lip balm** - Your lips may become very dry following surgery.

> **Body lotion** - Can be very soothing for dry skin.

> **Slippers** - Make sure they are the kind that you can just slip into. You will not be able to bend to pull up the back of a shoe. Take either flip-flops or rely on the hospital issue.

> **Nightgown** - If you take nightgowns, remember that you will have several IV lines attached to your hands or arms. Your nightgowns should be short sleeved. Most people utilize the hospital gowns, which come in large sizes. If what you are

given is too small, ask for a larger one. It is also a good idea to wear two hospital gowns at the same time, tying one in the back and another one that you tie in the front.

➤ **Camera** – Believe me, you will want to record your hospital stay! I am so glad that I had pictures taken of me in my bed and with my surgeon with all my flowers. They are a wonderful reminder of how far I have come.

➤ **Reading material** - Most people either sleep too much or are too affected by anesthesia to appreciate any reading material. If you do take reading material, a magazine will probably be your best bet. I was too groggy from the anesthesia and pain medication to read any heavy novels or even to do any crossword puzzles.

➤ **Family photos** – When your family can't be with you, pictures can be very comforting.

➤ **Clock** – A clock with a lighted dial or display is handy for when you wake up in the middle of the night and want to know what time it is.

➤ **Toiletries** - Hairbrush, toothbrush, toothpaste, makeup, etc.

➤ **A long handled spoon** - This will sound awful, but in the hospital you will need to go to the bathroom. Because of your incisions, it will be difficult to bend sufficiently to take care of your hygiene. A long handled spoon wrapped with toilet paper will help. The nursing staff is available to wipe you, and do it to patients all the time, but some patients are too embarrassed to ask for that kind of help. Hopefully, this will be one of the last indignities you will have to suffer because of your weight.

➤ **Talcum powder**-Your bedding can be more comfortable if you are completely dry from perspiration.

➤ **Comfortable clothes to go home in** - Your stomach area will be very tender, so you want to avoid anything that binds. Loose clothing is a must (preferably without a bra).

Hypnosis

Hypnosis is being used more and more in surgical procedures to help you to control what your mind perceives. Because pain is a perception, hypnosis can be used to control pain. Studies have shown that hypnosis and healing words said during surgery have a very positive effect upon the recovery process following surgery. It is important to understand, that the main function of hypnosis is to allow the body to better manage the pain and healing after surgery and does not take the place of anesthesia during surgery.

When a patient is under anesthesia, the auditory function is depressed, but we still never stop hearing, much the same as being in a hypnotic trance. The subconscious is in a very open state. Therefore, positive or negative words have 'a tremendous impact. Many surgeons speak to their patients during surgery, suggesting to the patient how well they will feel and how fast they will heal following their surgery. Patients receiving these positive words require much less pain medication during their hospital stay and recuperate faster.

Hypnosis and visualization are very powerful tools to aid your recovery and to help you to succeed.

Doctors at New York's Columbia-Presbyterian Medical Center studied patients using self-hypnosis who were undergoing coronary bypass surgery. In the study, 20 out of 32 coronary bypass patients were taught self-hypnosis and relaxation exercises. Those using these techniques, before and after surgery, showed significantly reduced anxiety, pain, infection and symptom reoccurrence, as well as better cardiac functioning after surgery, than the control group.

94

To find a hypnotherapist in your area, ask your therapist when you have your psych evaluation, contact the American Society of Clinical Hypnosis, 130 East Elm Court, Suite 201, Roselle, IL 60172 or visit their website at **http://www.asch.net**.

Visualization

Over and above healing statements and self-hypnosis, you can use positive visualization before and after your surgery. Take the opportunity every day of the month prior to your surgery, to do relaxation exercises. Sit comfortably in a chair and breathe deeply for a minute or two. Once you feel very relaxed, imagine your surgery and the positive, physical outcomes that you hope will be achieved. Imagine how you will feel and look after the surgery and see it as if it has already happened. See yourself walking briskly along a walking path or bicycling with your children. Imagine yourself walking into a regular clothing store and picking a size 10 dress and walking into the dressing room to try it on. See the dress slip easily over your hips and admire yourself in the mirror. See yourself visiting your family physician for a check up, getting onto the scale and seeing the number go to the weight that you desire. See your doctor's smile as he or she tells you that you no longer need your medication. Pick your own personal dreams and imagine them in as much detail as you can. Believe in your success and that you deserve to succeed. This can be a very powerful tool.

I practiced this technique twice a day before my surgery, as well as after. Not only did it help me to relax, it also kept me focused on my goal while building an inner excitement about my future. I had many moments of hysteria, but they would have been far worse had I not been using these visualization and relaxation techniques.

Anesthesia

More than likely, you will meet your anesthesiologist just prior to your surgery. You will have little or no time to develop any sense of whether or not you like or trust this person. You are probably so nervous about your surgery that, if you were like me, you wouldn't be able to identify your anesthesiologist in a line-up one hour after your surgery.

The mission of the anesthesiologist is to ensure that you are comfortable and free of pain during surgery. They determine what types of drugs and how much you are to be given. The anesthesiologist is also responsible for monitoring your vital signs, your blood pressure, oxygen levels, heart rate and respiratory rate. The objective is to have you maintain a level of unconsciousness just deep enough so that you are unaware of the surgery, but not so deep that your vital signs are affected. The anesthesia eliminates pain, awareness, and muscle reflexes so the procedure is easier for the patient, and allows the surgeon to operate more efficiently.

The mission of the anesthesiologist is to ensure that you are comfortable and free of pain during surgery.

As part of preparing you for surgery, a nurse will insert an IV into your arm or hand. Just prior to the surgery, you will be given a relaxant to relieve anxiety. During surgery, you will probably receive your anesthesia through a mask over your mouth and nose.

The drugs used during your surgery cause a temporary amnesia so that you have no memory of the surgery and the procedures immediately following the surgery. These drugs may also cause you to feel depressed. This usually shows up within a week or two after surgery as the last of the drugs wears off from your system.

Anesthesia poses particular problems for patients who have sleep apnea. When you are sedated, your muscles relax, including the muscles of the throat, which can cause an obstruction of your airway. If you have less of a respiratory drive, as sleep apnea patients do, narcotics can accentuate this problem even more. It is therefore important that you inform your anesthesiologist that you have sleep apnea so that you can be closely monitored, not only during surgery, but also in recovery.

An epidural anesthesia is another method that can be explored with your surgeon. In an epidural, a thin plastic tube is inserted through the back near the spinal column. A local anesthesia is administered through this tube. The drug acts as a nerve block to those nerves branching out from the spinal column causing a loss of sensation. The patient is conscious during the operation, but sedatives are given for relaxation. This is particularly useful for patients who have severe respiratory problems. An epidural can be used, not only for surgery, but also to control pain after surgery. With an epidural, the pain medication is administered to the lower part of the body rather than the entire body.

Breathing Tube

During surgery, you will be intubated. That means a plastic tube will be put down your throat to assist and insure your breathing during surgery. The tube is placed and removed while you are under anesthesia, so you neither feel it nor remember it. If you have a respiratory problem, the tube may be left in for a while after surgery, until the surgical staff is sure that you can breathe on your own. But this is very rare. Occasionally, the staff will have some problems putting the tube down your throat, so it is possible, but not probable, that you will have a slight sore throat from the ordeal.

I have no memory at all of my breathing tube. When I awoke in the operating room, all I remember is looking up at my surgeon and asking him how his little girl was (his wife had just had a baby). I experienced no coughing or gagging like you see in the movies. I may have done that, but the amnesia effects of the anesthesia blocked any memory of it.

Catheterization

Never having been hospitalized before, the idea of being catheterized terrified me. Catheterization involves the insertion of a tube into your urethra so that your urine output collects in a bag. The catheterization was done in the operating room when I was unconscious so I have no memory of its insertion. When I awoke from the surgery, I was grateful for the tube so that I did not have to get up to go to the bathroom. The catheter is a bit of a nuisance when you are trying to walk in the hospital. It is one more tube to have to maneuver around. The catheter stayed in for two days. By that time, I was more mobile and could manage to go to the bathroom myself. Besides, moving around is very important to avoid blood clots and pneumonia, the two nemesis of any surgery. When the catheter was removed, there was no pain or discomfort at all.

Fingernails

This seems to be a great concern of women as they are nearing surgery. I know it was for me. You should talk to your surgeon about what condition your nails should be in. Questions to ask would include:
> ➤ Should you remove all your fingernail polish?
> ➤ Can you leave it on all nails except for a few?
> ➤ What about acrylic nails?

The definitive answer is up to your anesthesiologist but your surgeon might be able to give you some guidance.

One way that your oxygen levels are monitored during surgery is via a clip on your finger. But some anesthesiologists and some nurses want to be able to check your nail beds for a visual confirmation of these levels. They can check your toe nails just as well. Check with your surgeon or his or her nurse.

I have acrylic nails. Although my surgeon and his staff did not feel that the acrylics were a major concern, I felt it was safer to remove the polish from all my nails and take the acrylic off of my index and middle fingers on both hands. If there was any problem during surgery, I didn't want anyone hindered by polish or acrylic.

Adhesions From Other Surgeries

Adhesions are scar tissue in the body that joins normally unconnected parts and are a common result of surgical procedures. If you previously had some type of abdominal surgery such as a gall bladder removal, the surgeon may have to deal with adhesions from that prior surgery.

Although rare, adhesions from the RNY surgery could cause the bowel to loop around, causing a bowel obstruction. This is a serious condition that requires another surgical procedure to correct.

Bariatric Bed

Bariatric beds are finding their way into more and more hospitals. They are larger beds that have controls that allow you to easily step out of bed by lowering your feet and raising your head in a slant, until you are in a totally upright position. Some patients love them, while others hate them. While they are very roomy and allow for easy exit out of the bed, which is a tremendous plus, they tend to have very compact and firm mattresses that hurt a lot of patients' backs. If your surgery was done with an open incision, having the ability to step out of bed, rather than go through the pain of rolling onto your side and pushing yourself up with your arm, is a great relief. However, when bariatric beds were first introduced, many nurses were not familiar with how they worked and couldn't instruct patients adequately. But, as more and more hospitals are being equipped with these beds, that problem should disappear. It is a policy of some hospitals that if you are over a certain weight, such as 350 pounds, you will automatically be assigned a bariatric bed. This is not only for the safety, ease and comfort of the patient, but for the benefit of the staff who are trying to get heavier patients out of bed.

Large Wheel Chairs

Be sure that you are provided with a large wheel chair as you are transported around the hospital. The regular sized chair will probably not be roomy enough. I know it wasn't for me. When I was brought a regular sized chair, before I got into it, I asked for a larger one and it was promptly delivered. You will be uncomfortable enough after surgery without having to squeeze into a regular wheelchair.

Blood Transfusions

Generally in weight loss surgery there is very little blood lost, making blood transfusions unnecessary. Therefore it is not necessary to store your blood in preparation for the surgery. Although some people have needed transfusions, they are very rare. Transfusions have only been necessary if there is a complication during or just after surgery.

Pain Control

Following surgery, many patients are given morphine to control their pain. This medication is self administered through a Patient Controlled Analgesia (PCA), sometimes called a morphine pump. This device is connected to your IV and will deliver a metered dose of morphine when you press a button. The PCA is programmed with a safety feature so that you cannot overdose. A measured amount of morphine is released each time you press the button, but you can only receive the prescribed maximum amount of morphine each hour.

While I used the morphine pump regularly, I especially appreciated it after I awoke from sleeping. I would feel a stab of pain and immediately push the button and would get almost instant relief. I would then be able to move; and moving is so important after surgery.

I found that the morphine alone did not give me relief from pain. My surgeon had also prescribed another pain medication called Toradol. This was periodically administered through my IV and was wonderful at controlling pain.

After surgery, if you are feeling pain, inform the nursing staff immediately so that stronger medication can be ordered for you.

Some patients receive their pain medication through an epidural. With an epidural, a small plastic tube is inserted through the back and into the spinal column area. The anesthetic put through this tube blocks the nerves that branch off of the spine and numbs only that area. Some patients experience nausea following surgery, and morphine tends to increase that feeling. Alternate forms of pain control are, therefore, important.

Caffeine

If you are a coffee or a coke drinker, you are accustomed to consuming caffeine every day. In fact, your caffeine fix might be very important to you. You might find it difficult to start the day without it. I would highly recommend weaning yourself off of caffeine prior to surgery, because you will not be getting any caffeine for quite awhile after surgery. If you do not wean yourself, you will wake up from surgery dealing with the pain of surgery and having to contend with a screaming headache from caffeine withdrawal. Not fun!

You should not be drinking caffeine after surgery either. It is very important that you drink a lot of liquids following surgery. You will be getting very little nutrition from food initially, so your consumption of fluids needs to sustain you. Caffeine is a diuretic, so it effectively dehydrates you rather than hydrates you. Not only can you not count your caffeine consumption towards your fluid consumption, you need to drink an additional 1 1/2-cups of water for every 1 cup of caffeine that you drink.

Caffeine is also an irritant and will be very hard on your new pouch. Try thinking of your new pouch as a baby. Would you give coffee to an infant?

Wills, Living Wills and Letters

Weight loss surgery is very serious surgery, as is any surgery. It is advisable when having any surgery to have your affairs in order. If you do not have a will, you should have one prepared for you that details how you want your personal effects and property disposed of in the event of your death. An attorney should prepare your will. But if attorney fees are not economically feasible right now, then there are several self-help books on the market, or available through your local library, to help you, such as The Complete Idiot's Guide to Wills and Estates or How to Make Your Will: With Forms (Self-Help Law Kit With Forms). There are several software packages that are also available to assist you in this, such as Quicken WillWriter and WillMaker from Nolo Press.

If you don't have a will, use this as an opportunity to have one prepared.

A living will is something completely different. A living will specifies what you want to be done to you medically if you are unable to speak for yourself, and who is empowered to make decisions for you. You will need to consider several options for your living will. Do you want to be resuscitated if you are terminally ill, or do you want to be put on life support if you have suffered brain damage? If you are in a coma and are terminally ill, do you want food to be withheld? If you are unconscious, whom do you want to make decisions about any procedures? All of this can be designated on a form that most hospitals can supply. Be sure that the hospital has a copy of the completed notarized form and that the person that you designate to make decisions for you is comfortable with your wishes and has a copy of the form. The <u>WillMaker</u> software, mentioned above, will also prepare a very good living will.

Many people having this surgery feel compelled to write letters to family members or friends that serve as a last goodbye. In some ways it forces you to focus on your relationship with that person, what your feelings are, and what you may have never been able to say. It can be very healthy and cathartic. I did not go through this exercise. On one hand I thought that it might be a comfort to my loved ones if something did happen to me. They would have a written record of my love for them. On the other hand my loved ones know how I feel. We tell each other every day. I also did not want to dwell that intensely on the negative possibilities. I felt that I had faced those possibilities and had moved beyond them with my decision to have the surgery. You will need to decide what is best for you.

Smoking

If you smoke, it is highly advisable to stop before your surgery. Let me put that another way. **Quit now!** You will be having major surgery and you will need your lungs to be in the best shape possible. Following major surgery, there is a risk of pneumonia and collapsed air-sacs in the lungs. You will be doing breathing exercises and coughing when you are in the hospital to help guard against these problems. Being a smoker interferes with your breathing at a time when you want your lungs to be as healthy as possible.

There are so many reasons to stop smoking.
Having weight loss surgery is just one more.

Being a smoker also has adverse effects upon your supply of oxygen during your surgery. A 1998 study done by the Medical College of Wisconsin in Milwaukee found that smokers undergoing surgery in which they were under general anesthesia, are 20 times more likely to experience problems with an inadequate oxygen supply to the heart, which can cause angina, the sharp crushing pain often felt by those having a heart attack.

Following surgery, it is also very harmful to smoke because smoking constricts blood vessels. A study done in 1995 at the Baylor College of Medicine in Houston found that smoking blocks oxygen from going to the site of the wound, severely slowing the healing process. This is an especially significant factor to consider if you are having an open incision for weight loss surgery.

There is one other smoking factor to consider. You are being given a new pouch, which is easily irritated. The chemical components of tobacco smoke can cause irritation of the pouch as well as ulceration. This is definitely something you want to avoid.

Prescribed Medications

Talk to your surgeon about the prescribed medications that you are currently taking and get his or her suggestion on when you should stop prior to surgery. This is especially important for medications that are blood thinners.

Herbal Supplements and Surgery

At least a week before surgery, you should stop taking over-the-counter medications that act as blood thinners. These include all aspirin and ibuprofen products as well as vitamin E.

What about all of the over-the-counter herbal supplements and vitamins that seemingly make us so much healthier? Although most people take some form of herbal supplement, as many as 70 percent do not report this to their surgeon. Herbal supplements can be very powerful and can have a profound effect upon how your body will react during surgery. At the 1999 annual meeting of the American Society of Anesthesiologists, the Society warned against the following herbal supplements. These should be discontinued at least two weeks prior to surgery to allow enough time for the effects of the herbs to leave the body.

➤ **St. John's Wort** – may increase or prolong the effects of some anesthetics and narcotics.

➤ **Kava-kava** – may increase or prolong the effects of some anesthetics and narcotics.

➤ **Ginkgo** – may increase bleeding by reducing platelets.

➤ **Garlic** – may increase bleeding.

➤ **Ginger** - may increase bleeding.

➤ **Feverfew** – may increase bleeding.

➤ **Ginseng** – may increase blood pressure and heart rate. May decrease the effectiveness of some anticoagulants.

➤ **Ephedra** – may interact with antidepressants or antihypertensives to cause increases in blood pressure or heart rate.

If you do take these up until the time of your surgery, be sure to tell your surgeon and anesthesiologist so that they can make any necessary adjustments.

Tubes

During and after surgery, your surgeon may elect for you to have a variety of tubes in your body. A breathing tube will probably be placed down your throat during surgery, and you will probably have a catheterization tube for urine. Often there is a Jackson-Pratt (JP) drainage tube placed in your abdomen to remove excess fluid from your abdominal cavity. There are two additional tubes that are rarely used, but you might encounter them.

Some surgeons will place a tube down your nose into your stomach. This tube is known as a naso-gastric tube or NG-tube. This keeps you from vomiting after surgery. The tube is placed when you are under anesthesia in the operating room, so there is no discomfort. Most surgeons do not require this, but some do prefer it.

A G-tube, or gastric tube is used for feeding. This tube is used much later if a patient experiences extreme difficulty with eating. It is rare that this is required.

Walk, Walk, Walk

Every day that you are in the hospital, you will be expected to walk three or four times per day, starting the day of your surgery. Your walking regimen will continue when you get home, walking around in your rooms and then continuing outside as you build up your endurance. The more you walk, the better you will feel. I have heard this over and over again and I experienced it myself. This will also signal the start of your exercise program for your new life. Walking is especially important because obese patients are at a high risk for blood clots in the legs following abdominal surgery. Walking helps to eliminate this.

Leak Test

If you have RNY surgery, you will probably have a leak test the day after surgery. This test checks your newly formed small pouch and all the bowel connection points for any leaks, which can be a very serious condition. A leak will allow food to seep into your abdominal cavity causing serious infection. A preliminary leak test is usually performed in the operating room to verify all connections prior to closing, and an additional test is usually required the day after surgery, before you can eat or drink anything. The second leak test is similar to an upper GI. You are asked to drink an unpleasant tasting liquid while you are x-rayed.

After my RNY surgery, I passed my operating room leak test, but failed my next day test. This is very rare; so don't let this overly concern you. The radiologist detected a very small spot that could have been a leak. The spot was gone by the next day. Leaks are very serious, but if you have an excellent surgeon like mine, they are manageable.

Breathing

Pneumonia is a concern anytime you are in the hospital and inactive. Collapsed lung air-sacs are also a concern. To guard against this, patients are given a spirometer, which is a little plastic device that measures your lung capacity and provides an incentive for you to exercise your lungs. I had to use the device four or five times a day by emptying my lungs then drawing air from the mouthpiece. This action causes you to fully expand your lungs. There is a small marker that you move to gauge your progress. As I used this device regularly, I was able to easily see my increasing lung capacity. I took the device home with me and used it for an additional week or two. A few months after surgery, I picked it up and measured my lung capacity again. I was amazed to see how much more capacity I had when I was fully recovered from my surgery.

Your Care While In The Hospital

Medical care has changed drastically in the past few years. Hospitals are hiring more licensed practical nurses and fewer registered nurses. The nursing staff has far more patients to care for. The pharmacy staff and nutritionists also have more patients that they are responsible for. For these reasons, if not others, you must be proactive about your care. Don't be afraid to question your care. If something does not sound correct to you, ask. If the answer does not make sense, ask to see your chart and your doctor's orders for the medication, procedure, treatment or food in question.

I highly recommend that your spouse, other family member, or friend, stay with you the entire time that you are in the hospital.

As soon as my surgery date was set, I called the hospital to inquire about a private room, and found out what was involved in guaranteeing it. I also asked about my husband staying with me. I followed up twice on this information to ensure that I did have a private room. Since I had a private room, my husband was able to stay with me during my entire time in the hospital. The hospital provided him with a folding bed and he never left my side. I was very fortunate that my mother was able to stay with our twelve-year old daughter at home during the five days that I was in the hospital. I did not have any neglectful care during my hospital stay; in fact my care was very good. But my husband was there to help me with my walks around the nurses' station, going to the bathroom, getting ice chips, helping me to deal with pain, and being a constant source of support and love. He was invaluable, and no doubt positively affected my recovery. I don't know what I would have done without him. I urge you to make these same arrangements. Even if it can be only for the first day or two, you will be very happy that you did.

C-Pap Machine In The Hospital

Those who suffer from sleep apnea use a C-Pap or Bi-Pap machine to ensure that their breathing continues while they are asleep. Check with your surgeon and your pulmonologist if you should bring this device with you to the hospital for use after your surgery. Although you may certainly still need it while in the hospital, there is a slight danger that the machine will inflate your stomach and intestines to the point that your stitches will be blown out by the force of the air.

108

If you do use it, your surgeon may require that the setting be some-what lower than what you may be accustomed to. Be sure to address this with your pulmonologist and your surgeon prior to your surgery.

Utilizing Occupational Therapy

Occupational Therapists work with people of all ages who, because of physical, developmental, social, or emotional problems, need specialized assistance to lead independent, productive, and satisfying lives. In the area of gastric bypass, Occupational Therapists enable the individual to reach independence through instruction on adaptive equipment and techniques for bathing, dressing, toileting, and homemaking. It is difficult for some people to bend forward or twist after bypass surgery because it puts pressure on their abdomen whether they had laparoscopic or open surgery. It may be difficult for some people to bend down or lift their leg up for socks, shoes, and pants. Occupational Therapy shows them how to use a "sock aid", "long handled shoe horn", and "reacher" so that they can put their shoes and pants on and off without bending forward or lifting their leg up. It also may be difficult for them to bend forward in the shower to wash their legs and twist to wash their backs. An Occupational Therapist will show them a "long handled sponge brush" to aid in washing their legs standing up and to wash their back with very little twisting. Another issue is toileting. It can be difficult to reach around to wipe after a bowel movement. Occupational Therapists have many different "toilet aids" which help the individual by extending their reach. If your toilet seat is too low it may be difficult to stand up from after your surgery and it may be difficult to stand for long periods of time in the shower or tub. Occupational Therapists also help with getting shower chairs, tub benches, and raised toilet seats as many different kinds exist. How long each person will need the above equipment will depend on their own comfort level and flexibility. If your surgeon doesn't automatically order occupational therapy for you and you are having any difficulty with independence, ask any of your medical doctors for an occupational therapy consult before you are discharged from the hospital.

21
Home From The Hospital

Everyone is anxious to be discharged from the hospital. Even though you rest better and heal faster in your own home, you will need help for a few days after returning. I mentioned this in Chapter 17, but it is so important that it bears repeating here. If you do not have any help at home and are completely on your own, speak to your doctor about staying at a rehabilitation facility where you will receive some care and assistance. Even if your stay is for a day or two or up to a week, this can be a tremendous help. You will be safer, feel more confident, and be more comfortable if you take your time recovering at a hospital or care facility.

You will need assistance when you get home. This is not a time to display your independence. Seek out and accept help.

The Trip Home

Ouch! You will feel every bump in the road. It will help if you have a pillow or large teddy bear to hold against your stomach for support. Be sure to take pain medication just before leaving the hospital. If you have a distance to travel, stop at least every two hours to walk around. Walking is very important to prevent blood clots.

Sleeping

Sleeping in bed can pose some difficulties. If you are accustomed to sleeping on your stomach, forget that for a while. Some find it painful to stretch out totally on their backs because it pulls on their incisions. If you are having this problem, you may find relief sleeping in a reclining chair. Some have gone as far as renting a hospital bed, but most do not find that necessary.

Another comfort for sleeping is a body pillow. These are pillows that are about four feet long that you can use to help position you in bed and to support your body as you are getting out of bed. Very comfy!

Drainage Tube

It is very common for patients to have a drainage tube inserted into the abdominal area during surgery. This drainage tube is known as a JP (Jackson Pratt) drain. This external tube is inserted into the abdominal area and drains any excess fluid. The tube has a bottle on the end of it that looks like a hand grenade or a "Huggie" bottle. The squeezed bottle exerts a small vacuum on the tube, causing any excess fluid, in the abdominal cavity, to be drawn into the bottle. If there is a bit of infection, it can drain out of the tube and the body does not have to deal with it.

The drain will have to be emptied and measured each day. The liquid will be a light red Kool-Aid color. If the liquid starts to look murky, yellowish or has a bad odor, this is a sign of infection and you must call your surgeon immediately. The bottle should never get full. If it does, it cannot create sufficient suction to drain the fluid. Therefore, empty it when it is about half full.

The drainage tube normally stays in about ten days and is then removed in your surgeon's office. The feeling when it is removed is similar to a hard menstrual cramp. The incision for the tube does not have to be stitched. It is steri-stripped.

The point where the tube goes into your body is covered with a gauze type bandage. You will be able to take a shower with this bandage on, but your surgeon may suggest that you take steps to cover it with some type of plastic. My husband wrapped several layers of plastic food wrap around me and held it in place with tape. It wasn't pretty, but it worked.

Activity and Returning to Work

You will be cautioned about lifting anything heavier than five pounds for the first week or two. This is extremely important advice to follow. You will also be advised not to drive for about the first week.

Returning to work will depend on the type of surgery you had, how strenuous your job is, and how well you heal. If you had a laparoscopic RNY surgery, have a very sedentary job, and are feeling very well, you could return to work in as little as two weeks. Generally, those having laparoscopic surgery return to work in two to four weeks. Surgery with an open incision usually requires a longer healing time lasting between four to six weeks.

Pain Control

Your surgeon will give you a prescription for pain medication for your use at home. One that is commonly prescribed is Roxicet, which is a liquid form of Percocet. Hopefully, your prescription was given to you prior to your surgery, so that your medication is waiting for you at home and you don't have to worry about filling the prescription on the way home from the hospital. Be sure to use your pain medication because it can make your life much more pleasant. You want to be sure to use enough so that you are not hindered from moving around. Activity is very important to your healing process. Moving around will help to prevent stiffness and avoid blood clots, which could be life threatening. But you do not want to take so much that you are feeling groggy all the time either. If you are too groggy from the medication, you will not want to be moving around. You should be sure to take your pain medication just prior to bedtime so you can sleep comfortably.

The amount of pain you will experience will depend upon many things. If you had an open procedure, you will have more pain than if you had a laparoscopic procedure. You will be dealing with the fact that your incision is ten inches long rather than five incisions that are 1/2 inch long. More muscle and nerve endings are cut in an open procedure and that will impact your pain level.

The amount of pain that you can personally tolerate will also impact how much pain you will experience. For whatever reason, some people tolerate pain better than others. If you have had surgery before, you should be able to judge where your pain tolerance level lies. Some people say that the surgery was extremely easy, while others think it was very painful.

You want to strike a balance with pain medication. Take enough so that you can move, but not so much that you are groggy.

The surgery process requires that the surgeon move internal organs to gain access to the organs being worked on. The amount of movement required will impact your pain level after surgery. For instance, if you have an enlarged liver, there may be pressure put on your liver during surgery that you will feel later.

Shoulder Pain

Many people complain of shoulder pain after they have had laparoscopic RNY surgery. In order to perform the surgery, your abdomen is filled with gas so that your stomach will be distended, giving the surgeon room to work. After surgery, this gas rises in the body as you become upright and the gas becomes trapped. This trapped gas can be very painful until it dissipates. Walking is one of the best remedies. If you experience pain in your shoulder, contact your surgeon. It may just be the trapped gas, but it might also be something more serious. If you still have your gall bladder, this is a common site for referred pain from gall bladder problems.

22
Possible Complications

There have been thousands of weight loss surgeries performed over the years. Techniques have improved and state-of-the-art medical care has helped to make weight loss surgery very safe. But complications are possible following any surgery, regardless of what type it is. Ten to twenty percent of patients who have weight loss surgery require follow- up operations to correct complications. I cannot stress enough, how important it is to report any problems to your doctor. If you have a persistent fever over 101 degrees, bleeding, increased abdominal swelling or pain, persistent nausea or vomiting, chills, persistent cough or shortness of breath, you need to contact your doctor right away. It is not necessary for you to determine if a true problem exists because that is your doctor's job to decide. It never hurts to ask and it could be very dangerous if you don't!

> *As morbidly obese patients, our susceptibility to serious complications during any surgery is increased.*

Here are some of the more common complications that can develop following weight loss surgery.

Blood Clots

Immediately following surgery, you are susceptible to blood clots forming in your legs. This is very serious, but if caught in time can be easily treated with a blood thinner. In fact, most surgeons automatically treat their patients with heparin. If left untreated or ignored, blood clots can cause death if they travel to your lungs or heart. Anyone undergoing abdominal surgery is at risk. Those who are morbidly obese are even more susceptible because of circulatory problems.

While in the hospital, you will probably wear a compression device on your legs, that pumps air in and out, so that your legs are constantly being massaged. You will also wear support stockings that help this process.

You will be encouraged to regularly walk in the hospital and at home so that your blood does not become stagnant, causing blood clots to form.

For a few weeks following surgery, if you experience any pains or cramping in your calves or notice any swelling in your ankles or legs, report this immediately to your doctor.

If you are particularly at risk because of a past history of blood clots, your doctor may want to insert a vena cava filter. This is a cone shaped filtering device that is put into your vena cava vein to catch any blood clots. This vein returns the blood from the lower half of the body to the heart. The filter is inserted through the main vein in the groin area and is moved up toward the heart. The procedure is normally done as an outpatient procedure, under local anesthesia or IV sedation. A catheter is inserted and dye is injected to aid in the filter insertion. The procedure is relatively painless.

Lung Problems: Pneumonia and Atelectasis

Pneumonia and atelectasis are risks following any type of surgery. Pneumonia is an infection that develops in the lungs. This can be very serious, because the infection could be coming from the gastrointestinal tract. Atelectasis is collapsed air-sacs in the lungs and is caused when there is a lack of movement of the wall of the chest, causing the tiny air spaces in the lungs to become squeezed. This is somewhat common and is not a serious condition.

You will be encouraged to cough in the hours and days following your surgery. While this is very good for keeping your lungs clear, it is not the easiest thing to do when you are dealing with an abdominal incision. You will also be given a breathing device called an incentive spirometer that measures how much air you take into your lungs when you inhale. This breathing incentive is very important to ward off lung problems. The nursing staff will know if you are suffering from any of these by listening to your lung sounds and taking your temperature. A fever is a symptom of pneumonia. Deep breathing and walking are two of the best deterrents.

You may also be receiving regular breathing treatments of medicine using the familiar "peace pipe" dispenser. The treatments come at all times of the day and night.

System Leakage

In gastric bypass surgery, a leak is a rare complication, but it does happen. When you swallow barium and stand behind an x-ray screen, the radiologist is able to track the path of the liquid and determine if it is staying in the pouch and then moving completely into the newly rerouted small intestines. If any of the liquid leaks out, the same thing will happen when you eat. If this is not corrected, the food or liquid that you ingest will leak into the abdominal cavity and cause an extremely serious infection. Normally, the leak will heal itself. If the leak does not heal, more surgery is needed to repair it.

Have an accurate thermometer at home.
Immediately report any fever to your surgeon.

Leaks are extremely rare. However, if one does occur and is ignored, death can result from infection. A generally acceptable leak rate for a surgeon is 2-3 percent of patients.

Symptoms of a leak could include left shoulder pain, a rapid heartbeat, increasing back pain, increased frequency in urination, increased frequency in bowel movements, and fever.

Another extremely rare, but very serious condition can occur when there is a leak where the small intestines and the pouch are connected or where the lower stomach bowel is connected to the bowel at the "Y" connection. When this occurs, fluid from the gastrointestinal tract, containing bacteria, leaks into the abdomen.

Gall Bladder

Whenever a person frequently loses and gains weight, they often develop gallstones and disease of the gall bladder. Gallstones are lumps of cholesterol and other matter that form in the gall bladder. Many overweight people have had their gall bladders removed prior to having weight loss surgery. If a weight loss surgery patient still has a gall bladder, a sonogram will check for gallstones as part of the pre-operative testing. During surgery, your surgeon will get a better look at your gall bladder and determine if it is healthy or should be removed.

Even after going through all of this, and your gall bladder is still with you after surgery, you could develop problems in the months ahead. About 30 percent of patients develop gallstones following gastric bypass surgery because of excessive weight loss. Some surgeons prescribe a bile thinning medicine such as Actigal, to be taken for the first six months. But because there is a 70 percent chance that you will not develop gallstones, and because these bile medications can cause weight gain, other surgeons do not recommend it.

Hernias

A hernia is a tear in the abdominal muscle that allows the intestines to bulge. This may be painful, or there can be no pain involved and the patient has no idea it is there. Normally you can feel the bulge.

Hernias are only serious if they become strangulated. This means that the intestines bulge through the tear and get squeezed. Incisional hernias will sometimes occur after an open procedure because surgery weakens the abdominal muscles. These incisional hernias are the most common long-term complication, occurring in approximately 10 percent of patients who have had open procedures. This is not a complication of the laparoscopic procedure.

Infection

Any surgical incision can become infected. It is especially important to note any foul smell coming from an incision. Also any milky, cloudy or dark drainage could be a sign of infection. Any redness or swelling may also signal problems. Report any symptoms like this immediately to your doctor. Wound infections occur in two to ten percent of patients and are generally, easily managed.

Bowel Obstructions

Following RNY surgery, scar tissue may form in the area where the small intestines have been joined. Scar tissue looks like cord or long strands. This scar tissue can loop around the bowel and cause a bowel obstruction, years after the surgery has been performed. A symptom of this problem is severe abdominal pain. This is a rare but serious complication that must be treated promptly.

Complications From the Pouch Size

Occasionally the pouch or the opening from the pouch to the small intestines will be made too small. This causes the patient to have a great deal of difficulty eating and to vomit excessively. While the size of the pouch will generally stretch a small amount over time, the opening to the small intestines, or stoma, can be stretched with an endoscope.

The reverse is also true. The new pouch or the stoma could be too large. The result is hunger and the inability to lose the desired amount of weight.

Nutritional Complications

The RNY surgery is successful because of two features – restriction and malabsorption. Restriction is accomplished by making the stomach very small. Malabsorption is accomplished by bypassing a part of the small intestines. Because the part of the intestines that is bypassed normally absorbs iron and vitamin B-12, it is vital that supplements be taken to replace these in the diet. If a patient does not follow the advice of his or her surgeon to take the proper vitamin and mineral supplements, then a nutritional deficiency may occur. This is especially true for women of childbearing age. Patients are typically required to take a multi-vitamin, iron, B-12 and calcium for the rest of their lives. By following these guidelines, no nutritional complications should occur.

Dehydration

Dehydration can occur at any time and for a variety of reasons. A very small number of patients experience vomiting, which can quickly lead to dehydration. If vomiting cannot be controlled, the patient will need to be admitted to the hospital to receive proper fluids intravenously, and to determine the cause of the problem.

Those who are newly post-op also have a difficult time getting in proper fluids because of the size of their new pouch. Water quickly fills the pouch, so you have to continuously sip to get in the required amount of fluids. Even those who are post-op for many months are susceptible to dehydration. If you have any feelings of tiredness or dizziness, try to determine if the cause is not enough fluids.

Medic Alert Bracelet or Card

Some patients feel more comfortable if they have a medic alert bracelet made that specifies that they have had gastric bypass surgery. Should you have a medical emergency and be unconscious and need to have a NG tube inserted which goes into the stomach, the medic alert bracelet will alert hospital staff to your altered anatomy. Medic alert bracelets are available at **http://www.medicalert.org**. The annual service fee, which includes a bracelet, is $35. Some surgeons provide a card to carry in your wallet that explains the procedure that you have had. My surgeon felt that it was totally unnecessary, but you may want to check with your own surgeon.

Deirdre

There are so many ways that my life has changed since my weight loss surgery. I am healthy, have had a successful weight loss and I would do it over again. As far as food is concerned, I would like to urge patients to be very careful with your choices. During your first year you need to make sure that you are getting tons of protein and very few carbohydrates. Once you start eating carbohydrates, they are addictive and hard to control. I did not eat more than 10 grams of carbohydrates or 5 grams of sugar per meal the first year. I know this made a difference in whether I lost 100 pounds versus 155 pounds. The surgery won't work unless you are willing to make permanent life-style changes, or you will go back to bad habits and the weight will return. The following is a list of the best ways that my life has changed since my surgery:

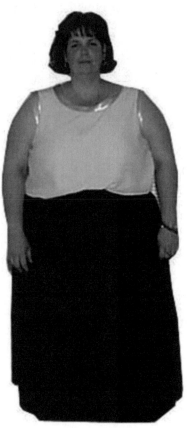

➤ I shop until I drop, I can't get enough clothes.

➤ I don't have pain in my knees or back anymore.

➤ I don't snore at night.

➤ I can eat almost anything. I just don't consume the whole bag!

➤ I don't eat as much as I used to. I get full very easily.

➤ I get asked out on dates for a change.

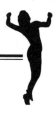

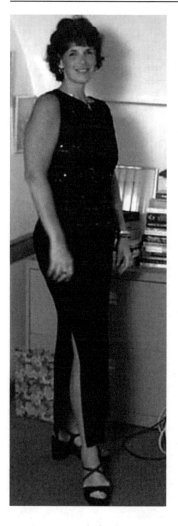

➤ I will be going skiing for the first time this winter with my children.

➤ I can not only fit in a movie theater seat, but I can also put my legs up Indian-style.

➤ When I drive, my stomach is no longer sitting on the steering wheel.

➤ I can sit in a booth at the restaurant, fit in the bathroom stalls, and comfortably fit in airplane seats!

➤ I can finally shop for pretty underwear.

➤ I was a size 32 and now am a size 12/14.

➤ People have stopped saying, "Oh, but you have such a pretty face!." I hated that one.

Sometimes I go by a mirror and have to stare because I still don't believe it is me. My inner person still has not changed. I am the Deirdre that I used to be twenty years ago, and she is something! I am not a pushover anymore. I'm not hiding behind my weight. And I'm not at the sidelines!

Deirdre

Jilda

On October 25, 1999, I had a Laparoscopic proximal RNY. On that day at 5'3" tall, I weighed in at 235 pounds and now, one year later, I weigh 125 pounds. Since that day, my life has changed in so many ways. I no longer fall behind, or become out of breath, when walking with friends. My thighs don't touch the sides of theater seats. I went sea kayaking for the first time and even wore a wetsuit (in public no less). My legs cross at the knees. I can play ball with my brother and nephew; not just watch

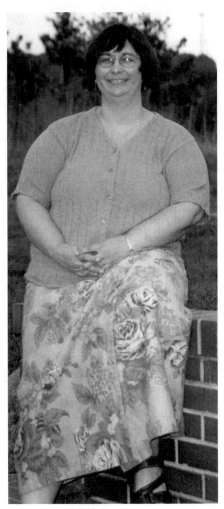

Before 235 lbs

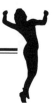

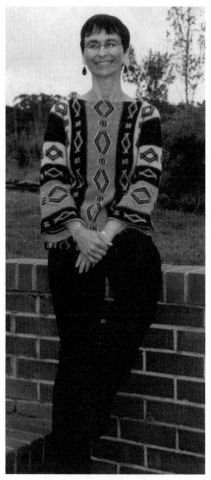

After 125 lbs

from the sidelines. Shopping for clothes is now an addiction. The pain in my knees when I walk up a flight of stairs is gone. There were times before when it was one step at a time. My fears of becoming debilitated, as I become older, have disappeared. But most importantly, I am more self-confident, out going, and have been told I smile a lot.

Jilda

Sue

Before the surgery, you are a fat person. You try to live day by day with everyone's judgment of you and they make the judgment without ever getting to know you. People look through you, around you or over you. I was not there; I did not exist. No one knew my struggle with food, but I had to eat to live. The prejudice against fat people is very accepted. They think it's ok because everyone does it. Society feels that it's politically accepted to look down on a fat person. I was not hired for jobs, because it's not the image they wanted to show. I was not offered a seat. I could not buy the clothes that I liked, because they were not sized that big. And everyone had a cure or comment for my weight problem.

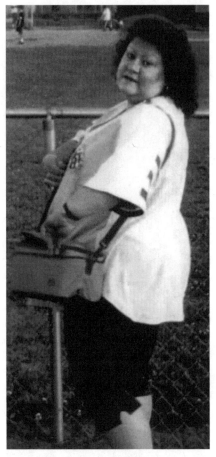

Before 250 lbs

Now people see me as the real person that I have always been. I feel that my current weight is what I should always have weighed.

126

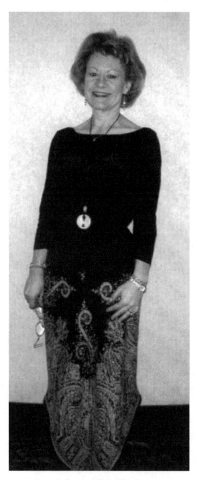

After 129 lbs

People now find that I am funny and fun to be around. I was before but they just didn't bother to find out. They say I am beautiful. I was before but they just didn't look. They say I am happier now. I was happy before, but it's just so hard to show happiness when people you deal with don't see or hear you. I always got the feeling from people that I was not worth listening to. People speak to me now who never did before. People are friendlier and nicer. Now I can sit anywhere and I fit into any clothes that I like. Yes, I am happier now, because the world around me wants to know me for who I am. I am worth listening to. It makes life so much easier and healthier.

Thank you Dr. Schauer for your skills and bedside manner.

Thank you Barbara Thompson for a voice. There are thousands more waiting to be heard. What will it be like with a world full of reformed fat people with a voice? Look out world!!!!!!!!!

Sue

Jennifer

The easiest way to describe the positive impact that weight loss surgery has made on me is that I now have a life and a future.

I first heard about weight loss surgery in 1998 when I was about 100lbs overweight. I already had many obesity related medical problems and a family history of early death from heart disease and diabetes. My own medical problems were getting worse and seriously affecting my health and quality of life. I felt that my life was in a downward spiral and feared an early death from obesity. I was only 43 years old at the time.

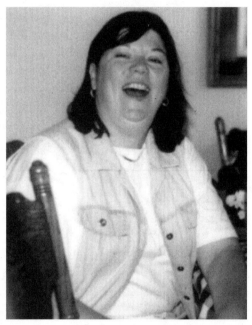

Before 243 lbs

I spent several months researching weight loss surgery. I was very concerned about any potential complications or side effects that could arise as a result of the surgery. I quickly came to the realization that there were probably no side effects or complications that could be as difficult to live with, as life threatening, or as life compromising as what I already faced with morbid obesity. So on 12/14/98, I took back control of my life and had laparoscopic Roux en-Y gastric bypass surgery. I lost over 100 pounds in the first nine months post-op, and regained my health and life in the process. I also went from a clothes size 22 to a 4/6.

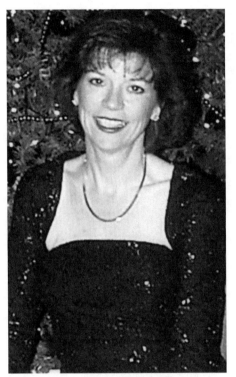

After 135 lbs

I understood that weight loss surgery was not going to be a quick fix or an easy way out. I knew that the surgery would prevent me from eating large amounts, but that it was up to me to develop healthier eating habits. So I spent some time learning more about nutrition. With the help of the surgery, I was able to develop a talent for selecting nutritious foods and eating them in sensible quantities. I believe I have built a foundation of healthy eating and good nutrition that will last me a lifetime. I could not have done this without weight loss surgery. It's what enabled me to get off the self-fulfilling cycle of unhealthy eating and yo-yo dieting. Weight loss surgery is often called a tool. How well you learn to use that tool is up to you.

The first year post-op can be an emotional and physical roller coaster ride. You need to make changes in your eating habits and lifestyle. For me, it also meant that I experienced a few side effects and complications along the way. However, these were minor in comparison to the obesity-related problems I had prior to surgery. Weight Loss surgery is not the answer for everyone, but it certainly was the answer for me!

Jennifer

Barbara

I am the author of this book. On Jan. 25th, 2000, my life changed forever. You know my story about how I arrived at my decision to have weight loss surgery. Here is my life now that I am 120 pounds lighter.

Walking past a mirror was always a painful experience. I just couldn't deal with my reflection. I must admit that I now enjoy looking at my new body. I turn to the side, stand up straight and look at my flattened tummy. It turned out better than I would have hoped and all without plastic surgery! The first time that I tucked in a top, I was so excited. That was a big step. Now, I won't wear anything that isn't tucked in.

Whenever the camera would come out, I was the first to run and hide. Now, I always seem to be asking my husband to take my picture. I like comparing my current pictures to my before pictures to reassure myself how far I have come. I still can't believe it is me.

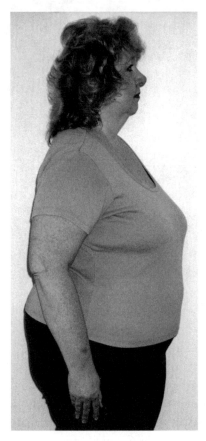

Before 264 lbs

Shopping for clothes has now become fun. I can't believe the sales that are available to "normal" sized people. I was never able to get

130

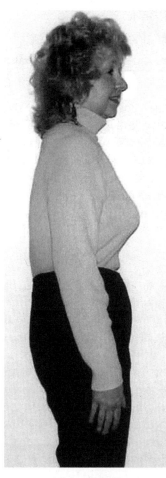

After 139 lbs

deals like this in the plus-sized stores. I bought a sized 10 pair of slacks that I would try on every month to see how close I was to fitting in them. The day I was able to pull up the zipper with ease, I went squealing to my husband. He shared my happiness because he knew how much it meant to me. Now that I am almost at my goal weight, I am rewarding myself buying my new wardrobe and enjoying every minute if it.

Physically life is grand. I have so much more energy to work and to play. I am not burdened with the constant pain that was crippling me. Now I can be as active as I have time for. I feel like I have to make up for many wasted years.

People have commented that my personality has changed. They feel that I am much more open and that my new self-confidence shines through. I know that I am smiling more at people and they are smiling back. I feel so proud of my accomplishment and proud that I had the courage to undertake this surgery. I chose to be healthy and happy. It was frightening at times, but there is no doubt that it was the right choice.

Barbara

23
Eating Guidelines Immediately Following Surgery

What you eat is what you get. It all comes down to nutrition. You have had your surgery, and now you need to know where to go from here. You will start out slowly and work your way through liquids, then soft foods and into solids. The entire time, you will be developing new eating habits in ways that you never have before. You are embarking on a true eating adventure. Sometimes the road will be difficult, but in the end, it will all be worth it.

Stage I - Clear Liquid Diet

Clear liquids will be started while you are in the hospital. The definition of a clear liquid is simply any liquid that you can see through. If you use this simple rule, you should be able to avoid any trouble during those first few days, as long as the clear liquids are sugar free or no sugar added.

Clear liquids include juices such as apple juice, broth, and herb tea such as chamomile, sugar free Popsicles and diet gelatin. During this first stage, you must be careful to drink enough fluid so that you don't become dehydrated. It is not necessary to worry about nutrition at this stage because hydration is your main goal. You should be drinking 2 or 3 ounces every 30 minutes. If you are nauseated during this time, check the sugar content of the juice you are drinking and consider eliminating the juice until your stomach settles down or try diluting it with water. If you are vomiting, switch to Pedialyte to avoid dehydration. Pedialyte also comes in Freezer Pops. Your doctor should be informed if you are vomiting so that you can be checked for any serious complications. Do not worry about drinking too much. You will be trying to work your way up to drinking 64 ounces of liquid per day. Be careful about the rate that you drink. Do not gulp; just slowly sip. Do not use a straw. You will be ingesting too much air if you do. Avoid all carbonated beverages – even diet beverages. The carbonation is too hard on your new stomach. Some patients have a difficult time drinking cold liquids; some cannot drink hot liquids. Stop drinking when you feel full, even if you have not consumed the specified amount. Take things very slowly.

The clear liquid diet lasts from one or two days to ten days to a month, depending upon the program of your particular surgeon. My surgeon recommends this diet for ten days following surgery. But make sure that you can tolerate the clear liquids very well before proceeding to the next stage. How fast you progress is also up to the regimen established by your surgeon. Keep in mind that you selected your surgeon because you had faith in his or her abilities. Remember that faith and follow the rules. Not following your surgeon's advice could put your health in jeopardy.

If you progress to the next stage and have problems with your stomach, go back to clear liquids. The liquid stage is always a safe haven. I had a very bad episode when I was about six months post-op, after eating whole leaf cooked spinach. It stuck in my stoma and caused me severe stomach spasms for 2 1/2 days. I gratefully went back to clear liquids for four days after that. I then added soft foods gradually until I felt confident that my bruised pouch and stoma could again tolerate regular food.

Stage II - Full Liquid Diet

A full liquid diet includes all of those liquids on the clear liquid diet plus liquids that you cannot see through. These liquids have more substance to them. They include strained cream soups. They may include milk; however try milk very tentatively. Many people cannot tolerate milk at this stage, so you may not even want to try it at this point. It is very common to develop lactose intolerance following surgery. This intolerance usually lasts only a short time, however. If you can tolerate milk, try adding dry milk solids to creamed soups for added protein. Your surgeon may also approve very thin mashed potatoes and very thin oatmeal at this point, as well as broth fortified with some baby food meat. Remember to add foods one at a time so that you can identify what may bother you. Many surgeons say, at this stage, that if you can sip it through a straw, you can have it.

Avoid orange juice, tomato juice and V-8 juice for now. They will probably be too acidic for your new pouch. You will be able to try these gradually in the months to come.

You may also want to try any of the low sugar liquid meal replacements such as Carnation Instant Breakfast, with no sugar added. There is not a sugar free variety and some people cannot tolerate the natural sugar from the milk in this. At this point in my progress, I tried a high protein powder. Big mistake! It made me very sick. It was not until I was six months post-op that I could tolerate high protein drinks, but I kept trying every one to two months until I got there. However, you may want to try the following: Mix 1 scoop of protein powder with 1 1/2 cups of Cool Whip Free. If it is too thick, add a little milk or juice. This is an excellent source of protein when you are on the full liquid diet and beyond.

You may want to experiment with making a smoothie. Use some frozen fruit like strawberries or peaches and whip the fruit in a blender with some cottage cheese, nonfat vanilla yogurt or some tofu. Try adding some high protein, low carbohydrate powder. Add crushed ice and some Crystal Light to the thickness that you like. Depending upon the sweetness of the fruit, add some Splenda or artificial sweetener.

At this point, it is not really necessary to be concerned about calories, but that question always seems to come up. You will be consuming about 300 to 600 calories per day. My surgeon recommended this full liquid stage from ten days until three weeks post-op.

The Full Liquid Sample Menu I received from my surgeon included:

Breakfast: 1/8 cup cream of rice or wheat.
                   1/8 cup diet pudding

Liquids Between Meals:
                   1/2 skim milk spaced over an hour followed by 1/4
                   cup low calorie beverage such as Crystal Light over
                   the next 30 minutes

Lunch: 1/8 cup cream of potato soup
                   1/8 cup sugar free blended yogurt

Liquids Between Meals:
                   Same as above

Dinner: 1/8 cup cream of chicken soup
                   1/8 cup diet Jello

Liquids Between Meals:
                   Same as above

Stage III - Pureed/Soft Foods

This diet includes soft scrambled eggs, cottage cheese, ricotta cheese, sugar free puddings, yogurt, pureed chicken, tuna or ham salad made with meat and mayonnaise, applesauce, tofu, pureed fruits such as peaches, mashed squash, and pureed carrots and green beans. You might also want to use baby food meats or potted meats. Mixing these with a little broth improves the taste. You may also have mashed potatoes, oatmeal, farina, grits or cream of wheat or rice. But because they are so high in carbohydrates, you will want to limit these. Regarding yogurt, make sure that it is the light variety that has approximately 100 calories per container. The regular flavored yogurt with the fruit on the bottom will be too high in sugar for you, and will probably cause dumping.

While this stage can seem very boring, with a little bit of imagination you can spice it up. By this time, after going through the liquid stages, you are feeling better and many patients get bored with such a limited variety of food. For instance, hummus and guacamole are both in this category and both high in protein.

If you haven't tried smoothies in the full liquid stage, or if they were too filling for you to enjoy, you may want to try them now. A good source of smoothie recipes is Smoothie Central at **http://www.quiknet.com/~mpenwell/smoothie.html**.

Your calorie level in this stage is typically 600 to 800 calories. Eat only when you are hungry and stop when you feel full.

Always eat your protein first. It is very important for you to change your eating habits to always incorporate the last sentence. I can't stress this enough.

Stop drinking liquids 1/2 hour before you eat and wait 1/2 hour after you eat to begin drinking again. This is important so that you are not filling your pouch with liquid and have no room for solids. You cannot get in proper protein this way. Drinking after eating causes food to be washed out of your pouch too fast for you to attain a feeling of being full and satisfied.

Do not try to see how much you can eat. If you feel full right away, stop. Some patients get discouraged from eating this extremely small amount of food, and mistakenly think that this is all they will be able to eat for the rest of their lives. This is not the case. Your capacity to eat will gradually increase over time. Therefore, take advantage of the small amount that you can tolerate now. If you are not hungry, and you are getting your proper nutrition, why eat? Enjoy it while it lasts!

My surgeon recommended this diet from three weeks to one month post-op. This is a maximum amount of food. I did not eat all of the carbohydrates in this menu and did not drink the milk. I initially had trouble tolerating milk.

A typical daily menu would include:

Breakfast: 1/4 cup soft scrambled eggs
                              1/8 cup oatmeal

Liquids Between Meals (spaced over 2 hours):
                              1/2 cup skim milk
                              1/4 cup fruit juice
                              1/4 cup Crystal Light

Lunch: 1/4 cup cottage cheese
                              1/8 cup pureed peaches

Liquids Between Meals:
                              Same as above

Dinner: 1/4 cup pureed chicken or baby food
                              1/4 cup mashed potatoes

Liquids Between Meals:
                              Same as above

Regular Food

You will be eating regular food after about one or two months, depending on what your surgeon advises. Do not skip to regular foods before you are permitted to do so by your surgeon. On a regular diet you will typically consume 800 to 1,000 calories daily. It is at this point that you will start to begin the important process of learning new eating habits. What you learn during these months will sustain your weight loss in the years to come. Simple practices such as eating only when you are hungry, eating your protein first and not grazing all day, will help you to live a long and healthy life. During these months, you can ingrain those behaviors into your pattern of dealing with food. Although you will be eating from all five of the food groups, it is very important to start with proteins first at every meal.

> *Don't rush yourself. Be patient and realize that you are not always going to eat this way. In a year, you will probably be able to eat almost anything, just in smaller quantities. So give your new system time to adjust.*

Food Journal

Start a journal as soon as you get home from the hospital. Record all of the details of your surgery and how you felt. Then day by day, record everything that you eat and drink and how you feel. This journal will help you immeasurably when you have any problems, and will make you more successful. Recording what you consume makes you more conscious of what you are doing. If you have a physical problem, your surgeon will want to know when the symptoms started. Your journal will have that record.

Recording everything that you eat and drink will help you when you are humming along losing weight with ease, and when you are not losing like you think you should. If you have a record of what you were eating when you were successful, you can compare it to what you are eating when you are not. If there is little difference in what you are eating now compared to when you were losing, you will know that your stalled weight is the result of a natural plateau and not because you are eating too much or the wrong foods. You can then more comfortably wait for the plateau to pass. Recording what you eat will also help you to not graze. It will cause you to pause before putting something in your mouth, if you know that you must record it. Further, if you record what you eat on a day when you throw up or are very nauseated, you will be able to see a pattern if it is repeated for the same food. Remember that initially, one day you may eat a food with no problem and the next day you may not be able to tolerate it. This is normal. It is all part of the adjustment process. Be sure to record your fluid intake and your exercise as well.

You will also want to record your weight and your measurements. Because your weight can fluctuate as much as five pounds in a day, most experts agree that it is probably better to weigh yourself once a week. I have never been able to do this. I always weigh myself everyday when I first get out of bed. I still cannot discipline myself to stay away from that scale! Weighing yourself less often than daily may help you to become less distressed when you hit a plateau. You won't be dealing with it on a daily basis.

Don't become obsessed with the scale. You will be getting smaller even if the scale is not registering a loss.

24

The Hunger Issue

Head Hunger

When you immediately come home from the hospital, you will be on a restricted diet, probably under orders to have only liquids. Although you will not be physically hungry, you may feel what you perceive to be hunger, but in reality is "head hunger." This hunger is as real as anything you may have felt before, however, this is your body's reaction to its first period of depravation. Your head is accustomed to your tummy being fed. This truly is not hunger, because your new stomach is extremely small and still swollen from the surgery. It is important to recognize this "head hunger" for what it is and abide by your doctor's orders to consume only what you have been advised to eat or drink. This feeling will very soon pass.

Lack Of Appetite

For the first 12 months, your stomach size and appetite are both very small which is the result of several factors.

First of all, your stomach is at its smallest. Over time, your new pouch will normally stretch a very small amount, but it will never be the size that the stomach was before. In fact, the new pouch is created using a region of the stomach that does not stretch very much compared to other regions.

Initially, your new pouch will be swollen from the trauma of the surgery. Your stoma (the opening between the pouch and the intestines) will also be swollen, which will cause food to stay in your pouch a little longer. Both of these conditions will act together to make you feel full for a longer period of time and will add to your feeling of being satisfied.

Also, after your surgery, you will have gone through many occasions when you have overeaten. You have taken the extra bite when you were full, eaten something that just did not agree with you or eaten too fast. All of these activities will make you feel sick, uncomfortably full or will make you throw up. Each of these activities works to turn you off of food, thereby affecting your appetite. You just don't feel about food the way you used to. This period normally lasts from six to twelve months and coincides with the period during which you lose the most weight.

It is hard to believe that anyone enjoyed eating food more than I did. I just loved it, and would consume huge quantities at every occasion. I enjoy eating food now, but not in the obsessive way that I did before my surgery. I have talked to many people who have had this same surgery and they feel this way as well. It is truly amazing.

Return Of Your Appetite

As you approach the 12-month mark, your appetite and the capacity that you can eat will increase somewhat. You will most likely continue to slowly lose weight for another 6 to 12 months, but you will reach a point where your food choices become very important again. You are at the point at which losing weight is not as easy as it was in your first year after surgery. This does not mean that you will gain the weight back, but it does mean that you will need to be careful.

At this point in your weight loss journey, you are probably within 10 to 30 percent of your ideal weight. At these percentages, you are considered a success in terms of your weight loss surgery. It is certainly possible to continue to lose until you are at your ideal weight, but it will take some work. Many people have reported that their appetite is as strong as it was prior to surgery. There is a very big difference however. The amount that you can eat is greatly decreased from what it was prior to surgery so that you are able to manage your hunger better. Your hunger may at times feel the same, but you cannot physically binge the way you used to be able to do. You may start to eat with the idea that you will binge, but you will quickly feel full. That is what will keep you from regaining your weight.

Your surgeon's job is done. Now it is your turn to utilize this wonderful tool to make this surgery a success.

The Internet site Cyberdiet.com **http://www.cyberdiet.com** is especially helpful when you are beginning to struggle again with eating issues. Remember that even though weight loss surgery is a very effective tool, it is your effort that makes that tool work. Within Cyberdiet.com you can build a nutritional profile that will tell you how many calories per day you can consume to maintain a particular weight, or how many calories to consume if you want to lose.

25

I'm Back On Regular Food, What Do I Do Now?

How Big Is Your Pouch?

Your new pouch will hold about one to two ounces, but it is sometimes difficult to get an idea of how much this is. Also, the size of your pouch is based upon your own physiology. The size has been likened to the size of your thumb or putting your thumb and index finger together as in the OK hand signal.

A method to check for the quantity that your stomach will hold is to do the cottage cheese test. Do not try this until you are two or three months post-op, so that you are not putting too much pressure on your stomach. Also, you don't want to check the size while your pouch is still swollen from the surgery. Take a full 16-ounce container of small curd cottage cheese. Eat the cottage cheese out of the container for five minutes until you feel comfortably full, but not so full that you are going to throw up. Leave the remainder of the cottage cheese in the container. Using a 16-ounce measuring cup, fill the cottage cheese container with water so that the water is taking up the space of the cottage cheese you have eaten. Check to see how much water you have emptied into the cottage cheese container. That is the size of your pouch. After doing this little exercise, you will have a better visual perspective of the size of your pouch.

Eating Slowly

Eating slowly has been the hardest behavior for me to master, and I am not there yet. It is very important to eat slowly. If you rush your eating, you will experience one of two things. You will either become nauseous or you will throw up. You can't sneak and gobble something down. Your new stomach is always on guard and will not let you get away with it. If you forget or try to cheat by taking just one more bite than you should, up comes your food.

Stop when you feel full. You can tell if you are full by feelings of pressure just below the rib cage in the center, a nauseous feeling, or pain in the shoulder area or upper chest.

Eating With a Baby Spoon and Fork

An effective way to slow down your eating is to use a baby spoon and fork. If you put only a tiny bit of food in your mouth, that will help to slow you down. Put the utensil down between each bite, chew each bite very well and then swallow. Before each bite, check to determine if you are full. If you are, stop eating.

Fiber

Foods that are high in fiber can be difficult for weight loss surgery patients to digest. It is difficult to chew high fiber foods enough so that they pass through the small stoma that goes from the pouch to the intestines. When these high fiber foods get stuck, you will experience severe cramping. One unexpected culprit is any fruit that has membranes, such as oranges or grapefruit. If you eat the fruit and not the membranes, you will be fine. Be aware however, that if you are newly post-op, the acid in citrus fruits may burn your stomach and the natural sweetness of any fruit may cause dumping.

Protein

Protein is essential to maintaining our health and is very important in our healing process. Even though beef and chicken are good sources of protein, they may be initially difficult for you to digest soon after surgery. Dark meat of chicken is easier to eat than white because white meat is so dry. Cottage cheese, hard cheese, ricotta cheese and eggs are also good sources of protein. Legumes (or beans) are also sources of protein, however they are very high in carbohydrates. I ate a lot of cooked cold shrimp initially, plus imitation crab and lobster on special occasions. I have never had any problems with any of these seafoods.

Tofu (bean curd) is an excellent source of protein, but not everyone enjoys it. Tofu is made from the curdled milk of soybeans that have been ground and then cooked. Tofu comes in the following densities: soft, firm, and extra firm. Tofu can be added to soups or it can be grilled, stir fired, braised or deep-fried. Because it has very little taste, it takes on the taste of any sauce or liquid that it may be in. An important advantage to tofu is that it is very easy on your stomach. It is soft, easy to digest, and is very easy to add small amounts to many of the foods that you prepare daily.

Eating protein first is such an important key to your weight loss success.

Strive to reach the point where you are eating 60 grams of protein per day. The body can absorb no more than 30 grams of protein in one meal so you will need to spread your protein intake over the whole day. Sixty grams of protein will be physically impossible to eat when you are newly post-op. Your small pouch just cannot hold enough to get an adequate amount of protein in. A way to accomplish this is to drink high protein shakes or to eat high protein bars, but the taste of these products is sometimes a problem. Many post-ops complain of a chalky taste to these drinks. But don't give up on them. I tried many protein drinks initially and each time they made me very sick. It was not until I was six months post-op that I was able to tolerate them. They have since become an important nutritional source for me. Carefully check the amount of carbohydrates in these products. A protein bar should have at least 20 to 28 grams of protein (or more) but no more than 15 grams of carbohydrates. If the bar has any more carbohydrates, it is nothing more than a glorified candy bar.

You should seriously consider using some form of protein supplement, in your diet daily, for the rest of your life, whether it is in the form of a protein bar or a protein drink. Protein is digested in the upper part of the small intestines utilizing the enzyme trypsin. Absorption of protein normally takes place in the first 12 to 18 inches of the small intestines. In RNY surgery, this part of your intestines has been bypassed making it more difficult to absorb protein. Supplemental protein is in a form that is easily absorbed.

Plateaus are a normal part of the weight loss process. Be patient. You'll start losing again.

Protein is a natural appetite suppressant and is essential for losing weight. When your body realizes that it is not getting the amount of sustenance that it is used to, it will go into a "starvation mode." This is the body's way of protecting itself when it thinks that there will be a lack of nutrition. Your metabolism slows to the point that even though you are eating a very small number of calories, you are still not losing weight and are at a "plateau." This is especially discouraging for those who are only a few weeks post-op. They are sure that they are the one person that weight loss surgery will not work for. They see themselves as failing another attempt at losing weight. This is far from the truth. They are just experiencing a normal body reaction to a drastic difference in the way they are used to eating. One of the ways to get off of this plateau is to boost your metabolism by consuming more protein. This convinces your body that you are not starving, and will be taking in nutrition. It is no longer necessary for your body to try to preserve itself through an extreme metabolic slow down.

Carbohydrates

Carbohydrates are the enemies of weight loss, whether a person has had weight loss surgery or not. No matter how much we were pre-pared for weight loss surgery, it is still a shock how little we can eat at one meal. We are used to a different relationship with food and often turn to our comfort foods, namely carbohydrates, as in the past. We find that, as we are able to tolerate regular foods, we are drawn to foods like cream cereals and mashed potatoes, which go down so easily. However, carbohydrates are not what you want to be eating at this point.

Your new stomach is very small and it is important to make the best use of the small space that is available in your pouch. In your heal-ing process, protein is vital for rebuilding cells. Therefore, eat pro-tein first. You will probably hear that over and over again from your surgeon, the surgeon's staff, and several times in this book. Also, remember that carbohydrates will make you hungrier. A small quan-tity of carbohydrates, such as 20 grams per day, is essential for good nutrition, however it is amazing and dismaying how many carbohy-drates are in foods that we would never suspect.

So what is so bad about carbohydrates? Depending upon the type of food you eat, different nutrients will be absorbed through the small intestines.

> From protein, your body absorbs amino acids.
> From fats, it absorbs glycerol and fatty acids.
> From carbohydrates, it absorbs glucose, a form of sugar.

Therefore, as you eat carbohydrates, you are putting sugar into your blood stream. The insulin in your body determines what happens with this sugar. Some is converted into energy, which is why athletes will load up on carbohydrates before an event. But you are not an athlete training for the decathlon, and normally do not need such a high boost of energy. Your body will use as much sugar as it needs to produce energy to do your daily activity, and will store the remain-der as fat. This happens with simple carbohydrates such as sugar, honey, fruit and milk as well as more complex carbohydrates such as flour, white rice and potatoes. If carbohydrates are not available in our bodies, then our bodies will burn stored fat for energy.

Also, when an excess number of carbohydrates are consumed, glucose is formed and insulin is introduced into the blood stream to deal with this sugar. The insulin causes our energy level to rise. When the insulin has dealt with all of the carbohydrates, our insulin level will drop and we will feel tired. This drop makes our body send out messages to get the insulin level back up. We therefore crave carbohydrates, we eat them, our insulin level goes up sharply, then drops, and the cycle starts again. Eating protein does not cause that increase in insulin. Our levels stay at an even level when we consume protein, so we do not have to deal with cravings.

If you are not losing, are nauseated, or are hungry, check the amount of carbohydrates you are consuming.

After surgery, try to keep your carbohydrate consumption between 20 to 40 grams (or less) per day. Some people are opposed to doing this, feeling that they had surgery so that they wouldn't have to diet again and counting carbohydrates is as bad as counting calories. Counting carbohydrates will teach you just how many carbohydrates are in the foods that you eat.

Become a knowledgeable consumer and check those nutritional labels on food packaging. You would be amazed at how many carbohydrates are in common foods that the American public eats every day. It is helpful if you buy a book such as Dr. Rachael Heller's <u>Carbohydrate Addict's Carbohydrate Counter.</u>

Food Values

There are many resources that you can use to track the nutritional values of what you are eating. A great place to look up food values is the U.S. Department of Agriculture's database. In addition to generic food listings, they also list some brand name products as well. Their web site is **http://www.nal.usda.gov/fnic/cgi-bin/nut_search.pl**.

Another place to find food values is the nutritional label found on the packaging of almost every food product sold in supermarkets today.

Water

Whether you have had weight loss surgery or not, it is important to drink at least 64 ounces of water per day. Nearly 75 percent of Americans know of the importance of drinking this much water, but only 34 percent actually do. Water plays an important role in many of your body functions, ranging from regulating body temperature, and oxygenating cells, to removing waste from your tissue cells. According to Dr. Donald Robertson, water suppresses your appetite and helps you to metabolize stored fat.

Your kidneys can't function without getting enough water. When they aren't working to capacity, some of their work has to be done by the liver. One of the liver's main functions is to metabolize stored fat into energy for the body. If the liver is doing the work of the kidneys, then it can't do all of its own work. The result is less fat being metabolized which causes weight loss to stop.

Water retention is another problem that drinking a sufficient amount of water can correct. It sounds like the reverse should be true, but if you are not drinking enough water, your body believes that it is not getting as much as is needed and it holds onto every drop. Consequently, when you don't drink enough, you retain more. This water is stored in the areas between cells and shows up as swollen feet, legs and hands. Taking a diuretic corrects the problem only temporarily. The body soon perceives the new threat and replaces the water the first chance it gets. The only way to overcome the problem is to give your body the water that it needs.

Water can help you to avoid constipation. When your body is not getting the water it needs, it looks for a source of water within the body. One place to draw upon is the colon. When your body draws upon the water stored in the waste in your colon, the result is constipation.

149

Some additional side effects of not getting enough water include fatigue, dry skin and headaches.

===
Water is another vital key to weight loss surgery success.
===

Your body still has the same requirements of liquid as before your surgery, yet your new stomach can hold only one or two ounces. Therefore, you must constantly be sipping to get in all of the liquid that your body requires. This means that you will have to carry a drink bottle with you at all times. Many people, who have been drinking large amounts of water pre-surgery, are surprised at how difficult it is to drink the suggested amount of water post-surgery. Many recent post-ops complain that water has a metallic taste to it. You can try putting in a bit of lemon juice, or drinking non-carbonated, caffeine free diet drinks such as Crystal Light. Any non-carbonated, caffeine free liquid counts toward your water requirement. It is not advisable to drink with a straw because you will swallow too much air into your stomach. This causes your small pouch to fill with air, leaving less room for fluid. If you are drinking coffee or tea with caffeine, you will have to compensate for the diuretic effects of the caffeine. Caffeine robs your body of water, therefore, you will not only be unable to count the coffee or tea toward your fluids, but you will have to drink an extra 1 1/2 cups of fluid for every cup of regular coffee or tea that you drink to compensate for the diuretic effects of the caffeine.

If you are eating a high protein diet, you are producing ketones that are harmful toxins to the kidneys. Large amounts of water are necessary to flush these toxins out of the body.

Watch your urine to determine if you are getting enough liquid every day. If your urine is dark yellow or slightly brown and has a strong odor, then you are not drinking enough liquid. Your urine should be a pale yellow color.

During hot weather, you should be extra careful about dehydration. Symptoms are dry mouth, lethargy, headache, dizziness, and extreme tiredness.

Another symptom of dehydration is cramps in your feet or legs. Water is essential to carry nutrients throughout your body. When you are lacking water, your extremities are the first areas affected, causing some people to experience cramping.

Water should be drunk cold if possible. It is absorbed into the system more quickly than warm water. Do not wait until you feel thirsty to drink. By the time you feel thirsty, your body has already started to dehydrate.

If you hit a plateau, check how much water you are drinking. This could very well be the problem. If you are not drinking 64 ounces, then you should be. Keep a pitcher of water in the refrigerator so that you can keep track of your consumption. Strive to empty the pitcher every day. You may want to drink more water earlier in the day rather than later, so that frequent trips to the bathroom do not disturb your sleep.

Splenda

Splenda is a low-calorie sweetener made from sugar that is not metabolized like sugar. It is slightly sweeter than sugar and is very stable so it can be used in cooking and baking. Splenda is being used as a sweetener in more and more products and may be ordered online at **http://www.splenda.com** or purchased in your local supermarket.

Drinking With Meals

Most people have eaten every meal, during their lives, with some type of liquid like coffee, tea, milk, water, or soft drinks. Drinking some type of liquid with your meal is a thing of the past after surgery. This is sometimes difficult for people to get used to. You should not have any liquid 30 minutes before and 30 minutes after meals. Here are the reasons. Your new stomach is very small and holds a very small amount of food. You do not want to fill your stomach with liquids so that there is no room for food. So you should not drink before meals. You shouldn't drink during meals because the liquid will tend to flush the food out of your stomach and you will get hungry faster. You shouldn't drink right after eating because you have eaten your food until your stomach is full. Putting extra liquid in now will cause you to throw up. Not a good finish for what was a nice meal!

Alcohol

Many people want to know if they can still drink alcoholic beverages after surgery. The answer is yes, with some restrictions. I had my first drink when I was about two months post-op. On rare occasions, since my surgery, I have enjoyed wine and martinis with no ill effects. I have also had beer and champagne, in very small quantities, but the bubbles have the same effect as carbonation. They expand in my pouch and make me burp. This is not good, especially if you have a toast to make!

Yes, you will eventually be able to drink alcohol, but not right away, and then only in moderation.

I would not try to drink any of the very sweet mixed drinks like Margaritas and daiquiris, etc. I am sure they would make me dump because of the high sugar content.

As a word of caution, remember that when you are newly post-op, you are striving to hydrate yourself. Alcohol will defeat that purpose; so drinking alcohol regularly is not a good idea. But on special occasions, it is certainly possible and most enjoyable.

You will probably not be able to drink the same quantity as before (assuming that at a social event you might have had two drinks). Your stomach can hold only so much. Also, the same rules about combining food and liquids apply. So if you are out to dinner and want a drink, try to wait 1/2 hour after you finish your drink before eating. Also, wait thirty minutes after you eat before having a drink so that you are not washing the food out of your stomach causing you to be hungry sooner.

Something that you want to be cautious of is that alcohol will get into your blood stream much faster now. Because of this, you will feel the effects sooner and more intensely. Watch this carefully if you are driving. You may have gotten away with having a drink and driving before, but you should definitely not try this after surgery.

Eating In Restaurants

Eating in restaurants can be a challenge. In my early days, post-op, dining out was not the adventure that it used to be. Before my surgery, I loved eating in restaurants and used them as an excuse to overeat. Now, however, I never walk out of a restaurant feeling guilty, like I used to. I walk out feeling satisfied and proud of myself that I have conquered the terrible food demon that has been with me all my life.

Initially, I tried to order the same things that I ordered in the past that usually came in large portions. I found this to be upsetting when I looked at what seemed to be a mountain of food in front of me that I was not able to deal with. Waitresses and waiters would always ask me, with concern in their eyes, if the food was satisfactory which was a nice way of asking what was wrong with my meal. I would take boxes and bags of food home, and never touch them. The experience of having a nice night out was not the same. I was miserable.

Children's meals do not provide the answer. These meals of hamburgers, spaghetti, pizza, and deep fried chicken nuggets, are poor food choices. Makes you wonder why we feed these meals to our children. Some restaurants will offer senior portions that are merely smaller portions of adult food, which is a start, but rarely do they approach the variety of a normal menu. Appetizers or soup offer a good alternative. One of my favorite "entrees" is shrimp cocktail. I also enjoy a small crab cake appetizer as a meal. And most soups are good fillers. I have also ordered a regular meal and asked the waitress to not even bring the salad, but to immediately box it with the dressing of my choice. Then when I am served my entrée, I eat half of the protein, a forkful of the carbohydrate and take the rest home along with the salad that was not even served to me.

Another problem of a full sized meal is staring at the remaining food and feeling overwhelmed. To solve this problem, I have the server box the remainder as soon as I am finished. I have less temptation to pick and possibly over eat to the point of throwing up.

Many surgeons will provide their patients with a card to use in restaurants that explains that their patients have had stomach surgery and are able to eat only very small amounts. These cards request that patients be permitted to order and pay for child-sized portions. It is up to the restaurant if they want to honor these cards or not. If your surgeon does not provide these cards, you can print them out from the following link, **http://www.obesityhelp.com/morbidobesity/restaurantcard.html**.

Be very careful about trying something new in public. If the food does not agree with you, you could be in a bit of trouble. If you do need to try something new because it is a set menu, try a small piece and see how it goes down. Do not overdo it. Also, be careful about eating too much or too fast. In a social setting, we can get carried away and not remember our new training – chew, chew, chew and stop when we are full. I must admit I have had to walk hurriedly to the ladies room on more than one occasion because of that.

Get used to take-out containers. You will always have a nice lunch the next day.

Here is one last tip about eating in a restaurant that should allow you to feel that you are having a pleasant experience. Order from the menu based on what you would like to eat (within the guidelines of healthful food) and don't worry about the quantity that is served. You can always take home what you don't eat and enjoy it again for lunch. Try to order in smaller quantities, if possible, but don't opt for something else just because the quantity is less. If you deprive yourself of the things that you are able to eat just because there is too much, you will not be totally happy with your surgery and be very discouraged.

26
Vitamin Supplementation

Following surgery, the issue of taking vitamins takes on a whole new importance compared with prior to your surgery. Before surgery, you may have just grabbed any vitamin that happened to be on sale at your local grocery store without putting much thought into it. And the issue whether you took vitamins or not, may not have mattered that much. Well that was then and this is now!

Vitamins play an essential role in how you feel not only in the months following weight loss surgery, but for the rest of your life. Prior to surgery, you probably took vitamins, but not with any sense of urgency. Your only reason for taking them may have been because that is what people normally do. But your body is different now and it is important that you consider vitamins and how they affect your health in a whole new way.

Making matters worse is the fact that the better the vitamin, the larger the pill. Many patients fear swallowing large pills, apprehensive that the pills will become stuck in their stoma. Additionally, after your surgery, your sense of taste is altered and distorted for a few months. Therefore liquid or chewable vitamins that might have been tolerable prior to surgery are positively intolerable after. Unfortunately the result is often that patients avoid taking any vitamins at all, because they cannot find a solution that is right for them.

I know this because I went through the exact same thing. I thought before my surgery that I had my vitamin issue under control. That was the least of my worries. I was just worrying about surviving the surgery, not what vitamin I was going to take. But after I recovered, I could feel that I really needed help from vitamins to start feeling as good as I looked. I then went on a 2-year search for a vitamin solution. I tried the liquid and children's chewable vitamins. I tried the caramel calcium chews that did no good at all, except taste good and the calcium that caused me to be constipated. And then I just stopped taking anything and was getting increasingly more tired. I was lucky that I finally found a total solution with the Isotonix line of vitamins.

The lower part of the stomach and the upper part of the small intestines normally play an important role in the absorption of vitamins and minerals. Because these areas are bypassed after RNY surgery, it is important for patients to take vitamin supplements regularly for the rest of their lives. However, not all vitamins are created equal. Therefore for optimum benefit, you need to keep some things in mind.

Problem With Pills

When taking vitamin pills, manufacturers rely on the fact that you have extremely harsh gastric juice in your stomach in order to break down pills for absorption. However, consider the following chart which shows the absorbency rate of supplements for a person with a **normal** stomach and **normal** digestion. This chart refers to people with far greater ability to digest compared to RNY patients.

Pills	3% to 20% absorbed
Gel Caps	15% to 35% absorbed
Chewable	35% to 50% absorbed
Liquid	50% to 75% absorbed
Isotonic	90% to 98% absorbed

Pills and Gel Caps- During normal digestion, supplements in pill and gel cap form must sit in your stomach for a long time until the gastric juice dissolves them enough to be absorbed. With our altered anatomy, we do not have sufficient time nor sufficient gastric juice for pills to break down completely in our new pouch, thus we have the great potential for supplements in pill form to not be absorbed at all. There is the additional problem of pills becoming lodged in the opening between the pouch and the small intestines. This blockage can be extremely painful. And it seems the better the vitamin pill, the larger it is.

Chewable Vitamins – Chewable adult vitamins are difficult to find and expensive without a prescription. With chewable vitamins there is the additional problem of taste.

Liquids - Unfortunately the liquid variety of vitamins while having a higher absorption level, tend to taste terrible.

Isotonic – This is by far the best source of vitamin and calcium supplementation for everyone, regardless of whether they had bariatric surgery or not.

If a substance is isotonic, that substance has the same concentration as our own body fluids such as our tears and is highly absorbable to the tissues of the body like an IV fluid.

Before anything in the stomach can be absorbed, the gastric juices of the digestive system must break it down to create a solution that is isotonic. This isotonic fluid is required to pass through the tissues of the intestines into the bloodstream. This is a problem for gastric bypass patients because most of the gastric juices are isolated from what is in the pouch. If a vitamin or calcium pill is in the pouch, very little dissolving occurs which results in very little nutritional benefit.

When a nutritional supplement is taken as an isotonic solution, the stomach or pouch does not have to perform any digestion at all. The solution is already in the proper solution necessary to achieve the maximum absorption at the fullest potency.

What to Take

Your surgeon will advise you specifically according to your blood work and how you feel, but generally these are the vitamins that most post-op patients take:

Multi-vitamin - Take a good general multi-vitamin, one that provides a minimum of 100% of the essential vitamins and most minerals. A chewable children's vitamin is not a good substitute. Obviously they are not meant for the nutritional needs of adults. There is a chewable adult vitamin that is available by prescription only. It is a prenatal vitamin and is called Natachews. For a non-prescription vitamin, the best I have found is the Isotonix Multivitamin. It comes in powdered form, mixes with water and is almost completely absorbed within 5 minutes.

B-12 – There are three methods of taking Vitamin B-12: by ingestion (swallowing), monthly injections and sublingually (under the tongue). If you select any of the oral methods, you should receive 500 micrograms daily. Vitamin B-12 is essential to keep your nervous system working well and for normal red blood cell development. B-12 can be found in animal foods, but not plant foods. B-12 is normally absorbed in the part of the intestines that is bypassed, which is why a B-12 supplement is necessary for RNY patients.

The amount of B-12 that you absorb from food and oral supplements depends upon a chemical substance called the intrinsic factor which is produced in the lining of the stomach when stimulated by food. The amount of intrinsic factor available after RNY surgery varies from patient to patient. Some patients after gastric bypass surgery continue to produce some intrinsic factor in the stomach that will help them in absorbing B-12. Others do not and their B-12 levels must be treated more aggressively. You will need to take some form of B-12 supplementation. How much you need will depend upon your B-12 levels which should be checked annually.

After years of low levels of B-12, patients can develop pernicious anemia which can damage the central nervous system and spinal cord. Be sure not to neglect taking B-12 supplements.

Calcium – Calcium is critical to bone growth, the regulation of blood pressure, and blood clotting as well as muscle and nerve control. People aged 19 to 50, need a calcium intake from all sources of 1,000 mg of calcium per day and those older than 50 need 1,500 mg per day.

The best source of calcium comes from natural food. The following are some common sources of calcium found in the food you eat:

Milk, 1 cup	295 mg
Yogurt, 1 cup	450 mg
Cottage cheese, 1 cup	155 mg
Cheese, 1 oz.	205 mg
Broccoli, 1 cup	180 mg
Salmon, 3 oz.	190 mg
Almonds, 3 oz.	198 mg
Tofu, 1 cup	130 mg

Calcium is found in most foods and a good nutrition book will list the levels for you. Once you become accustomed to looking for calcium amounts in food, you will get a sense of how much calcium you normally eat. When selecting foods, choose those with added calcium. However, even if you believe that you are eating 1,000 to 1,500 mg of calcium daily, it is still necessary to take calcium supplements, because the amount of calcium that you eat and the amount that is available to be used by your body are two different things.

Osteoporosis is the result of a lack of sufficient calcium which causes a thinning of the bones. Unfortunately there are no easily identifiable symptoms of osteoporosis, until the painful tragedy of a broken bone results.

The calcium in your body that keeps your bones thick and strong is like a savings account. The calcium that you get from food and calcium supplements is like a checking account. Your body requires calcium through the course of a day and it takes it from the calcium that you take in each day from food and supplements (your checking account calcium). When you aren't taking in enough calcium and your calcium checking account doesn't have enough in it, your blood pulls calcium from your bones (the savings account). The body does this automatically and does not report to you how much overdrawn your checking account calcium may be and how depleted and thin your bones are becoming.

One of the reasons that osteoporosis is such a problem is that we are eating fewer foods rich in calcium. In my own situation, all of my adult life I would drink a glass of iced tea or diet Coke with dinner. I wouldn't even think of having a glass of milk. And now that I am post-op I don't drink anything at all with dinner. Also for the first few months following RNY surgery, it is not uncommon for patients to develop lactose intolerance. This usually disappears after a few months.

The major reason however that osteoporosis is such an issue with RNY patients is because the typical ways of absorbing calcium from supplements is interfered with by our new anatomy. While osteoporosis is a risk for anyone as they age, with RNY patients it is a major concern and taking the right calcium supplement is mandatory.

Calcium supplements come in many different forms and come in many different kinds of calcium. The common types are calcium carbonate, calcium citrate, calcium phosphate, calcium lactate and calcium sulfate. When selecting the form of calcium to take, you need to consider the following factors:
1. The amount of elemental calcium available in each form and
2. How easily we as weight loss surgery patients with our altered anatomy can absorb that type of calcium and
3. The effectiveness of the delivery system such as pill, chewable or isotonic that the calcium gets into our blood stream.

Elemental calcium is the actual amount of calcium available in each calcium product that your body is able to absorb under perfect circumstances. Calcium carbonate provides 40% of elemental calcium, so if you were to take 1,000 mg of a calcium carbonate, you would be receiving only 400 mg of usable elemental calcium under ideal conditions. Calcium citrate provides 21% of elemental calcium.

Therefore if you were taking 1,000 mg of calcium citrate, you would be receiving 210 mg of usable elemental calcium.

Calcium is very finicky when it comes to combining with other substances. For instance you should not take an iron supplement at the same time as you take calcium. The iron will prevent the calcium from being absorbed. The same holds true if you are taking a multivitamin that contains a large percentage of iron. Do not take that the same time as your calcium. Other substances that naturally occur in food can inhibit calcium absorption. Spinach for example is high in calcium, but because spinach contains oxalic acid, which prevents the absorption of calcium, spinach is not a good source of calcium. Our bodies are also limited by the amount of calcium that we can absorb at one time which is generally no more than 500 mg of elemental calcium in a single dose. Therefore, it is important to split doses throughout the day.

The other consideration in choosing a calcium supplement is absorption. Although there is more elemental calcium available in calcium carbonate, this form of calcium normally requires gastric juice to be absorbed, something RNY patients have very little of. Therefore, taking calcium carbonate in any form that requires the body to digest it will result in poor absorption.

Another form of calcium to consider is calcium citrate. When taken in a pill form, it is optimally absorbed on an empty stomach and does not require gastric acid. Magnesium in a 2:1 ratio or twice the amount of calcium as magnesium, as well as vitamins C and D to aid absorption should be included in the formulation. If you want to take calcium in a pill or non-isotonic form, calcium citrate is better than any of the calcium carbonate forms. The advantage to calcium citrate is that it does not require gastric juice for absorption. The disadvantages are that it is low in elemental calcium and people often report resulting digestive problems, such as constipation.

The optimum form of calcium product is available in an isotonic formula which you drink. Isotonic means that the liquid mimics or resembles our own body fluid such as our tears and is rapidly absorbed like an IV fluid. Because the body more readily absorbs an isotonic liquid, it is absorbed into your system within 5 minutes. Isotonic formulas are the wave of the future for all vitamin supplements as more people realize the cost and health benefits of an isotonic product that has a higher absorbency compared to a pill that passes through the body with a very low absorbency rate. Isotonic calcium ionizes calcium molecules and releases them so that all of the calcium can be absorbed without requiring gastric juice to be present. This allows you to take forms of calcium that are much higher in elemental calcium. The isotonic calcium, which comes in a powdered form, when mixed with water becomes ionized. Therefore everything that used to occur in our stomach regarding calcium now occurs in our cup even before drinking it.

All forms of calcium are not created equal and neither are all delivery systems!

There are several antacid products on the market that claim to be good sources of calcium. Many people take these products feeling secure that they are giving their bodies the nutrients that will allow them to avoid osteoporosis in the future. Although these products are very good as antacids, I would not recommend them for the purpose of getting your daily calcium. The form of calcium used in these products is calcium carbonate, which is formulated with antacid ingredients. If your reason for taking this combination is for your calcium intake, you have a BIG problem. As stated earlier, calcium carbonate not in an isotonic formula needs gastric acid to be absorbed. These products, by their very nature of being antacids, *prevent* absorption. Since we have little or no gastric juice in our stomach pouch, antacids, as a calcium supplement, are useless for bypass patients. Calcium also needs vitamin D to aid absorption, which is not present in antacid formulations.

Many people take caramel calcium chews because they are yummy, do not cause dumping and contain vitamin D. However, the form of calcium used in these is also calcium carbonate. These chews might be sufficient for people who have not had bypass surgery and have better absorption, but because of our reduced absorption ability, and lack of gastric juice, it is not what we should take. In my early days post-op, these chews were my breakfast treat. I just loved those delicious little caramels! I no longer take them because I worry about my ability to absorb the calcium carbonate and the resulting greater chances of osteoporosis. I might take them for a caramel treat, but not to supply my calcium needs.

Do not take calcium that contains bone meal, dolomite, or oyster shells because they may contain lead and other toxic substances.

We tend to think that our bones are inert or dead material, but they are not. Bone tissue is living and growing material that reacts to what we eat, how well we absorb what we eat, and how we exercise. When we were heavier, bone density was not as much of a problem. Nature provides that as you get larger, your bone density increases to support your weight. Now that we are getting to be a normal size post-operatively, our bones become less dense and osteoporosis becomes more of a concern.

Both males and females should be concerned about getting the proper amount of calcium, but this becomes critical for those of us who are losing weight. Dr. Edward Mason, considered to be the father of weight loss surgery, in the Fall 2000 issue of the IBSR Newsletter, expressed his concern that not enough is known about the link between bypass surgery and osteoporosis. He states that osteoporosis is difficult to diagnose during early stages when it is easiest to prevent. He emphasizes the importance of taking calcium as a preventive measure against this disease. Be good to those bones by taking calcium daily and in the correct form.

Iron - It is difficult to find the right iron to take because of our new absorption problems. You should take ferrous fumarate or ferrous gluconate. Do not take ferrous sulfate as it tends to cause gastric irritation. Iron should be taken on an empty stomach with vitamin C. In order for iron to be absorbed, it cannot be taken with your calcium supplement. In fact, you should not take iron within one hour of eating cheese, yogurt, milk, eggs, spinach, tea, coffee, whole grain breads, cereals and bran. I currently take a prescription iron pill called Niferex 150 Forte because my blood work showed that despite taking the over-the-counter iron pills, my iron levels were low. It is very easy on the stomach and has helped my energy level tremendously.

If you are eating protein and drinking water and are still feeling tired, have your blood levels checked. You might be deficient in iron or B-12.

When you are deficient in iron, you are anemic. Symptoms are light-headedness, weakness, dizziness, and in severe cases, your pulse rate goes up and your blood pressure goes down. Without sufficient iron, the body can't manufacture enough new red blood cells packed with hemoglobin, the red-cell protein that transports oxygen. Your body will be starved for oxygen.

Many people complain about being constantly cold following surgery. While this may be the result of losing a thick layer of fat that kept you warm, it may also be caused by a lack of iron in your diet. Have your iron levels checked.

One of the most easily absorbed sources of iron comes from lean red meat. Dietary iron comes in two forms, heme and non-heme. Heme iron forms hemoglobin and comes only from animal sources and is easily absorbed by the body. Non-heme iron is found in plants and is not easily absorbed.

Other Supplements to Consider

Although a multi-vitamin, calcium, B-12, and iron are the vitamin regime you need to follow, there are other supplements that you might want to consider for optimum health. I started taking these supplements more than 2 1/2 years after my surgery and they have made a tremendous difference in how healthy I feel and the energy I have.

Antioxidant – We must breathe to live, but the very act of breathing causes a process in our bodies called oxidation. We have seen evidence of this same process in nature with the browning of a cut apple or the rusting of metal. The process of oxidation in our bodies is the result of free radicals. A free radical is a molecule in the body that has an unbalanced charge. Free radicals energize our bodies, but an over abundance are harmful. Free radicals occur by the millions, as our bodies are subjected to preservatives in food, UV rays from the sun, sources of radiation such as cell phones and microwaves, pollution and chemicals in our environment and even excessive exercise. All of this extra exposure leads to the aging process as our bodies break down. Antioxidants fight against excessive free radicals in our bodies, fight disease and slow the aging process. The best source of antioxidants is something called oligomeric proanthocyanidins (OPC) especially those derived from grape seed, pine bark and red wine. Taking an OPC can help an amazing array of diseases including diabetes, high cholesterol, allergies, heart disease, cancer, auto immune diseases, and inflammatory diseases. No one should be without an antioxidant.

Please note however, that antioxidants have blood thinning properties, therefore if you are taking these before your surgery, you will want to stop 14 days prior to surgery and then start again after your surgery.

Digestive Enzymes - Enzymes allow your body to digest and absorb food. Your immunity, your vitality and longevity depend upon your enzyme production and the enzymes we get from raw food or from supplements. Our altered digestive system compromises the amount of enzymes our body has available. Cooking or processing food destroys enzymes, so our diet allows for little enzymes. So it is wise to take a good enzyme supplement.

166

One function of enzymes is to aid the body in the digestion and burning of fat for energy so that fat does not accumulate in the body. An interesting study was done by veterinarians who fed one group of animals enzyme-rich raw potatoes and another group of animals enzyme-deficient cooked potatoes. The animals that ate the cooked potatoes gained weight rapidly. The animals that ate the raw potatoes did not.

Because very little of our food is eaten raw, digestive enzyme supplements are an important and excellent way to ensure that sufficient digestive enzymes are in your body so that you will burn the maximum amount of fat after your surgery, boost your immunity, have friendly bacteria in your colon and have the energy you need by helping you to absorb all the nutrients in your food.

Visit my website http://www.wlscenter.com/Vitamins.htm or call our office (877) 440-1518 toll free for more information about these and other vitamin supplementation.

27
Initial Problems

Why Does This Taste Different?

Many bypass patients report that their tastes change after surgery. Foods that tasted good before, just don't taste the same, or have the same appeal, after surgery. Sweets may just taste too sweet now, and there is a study that supports that phenomenon. Dr. Jean Burge, et al at Ohio State University, tested taste sensitivity to sweets and bitter foods on 14 RNY patients in a study reported in the <u>Journal of the American Dietetic Association</u>. The team tested taste sensitivity prior to surgery, six weeks after surgery, and twelve weeks after surgery. They used a number of people on a very low calorie diet as a control group. The surgery group had a dramatic increase in sensitivity to sweets after surgery, at both the six and twelve week intervals. The control group on the very low calorie diet had no change in sensitivity to sweets. When the sensitivity to bitter taste was tested, there was no difference in either group. Researchers noted the dramatic difference in the sensitivity to sweets in the surgery group and concluded that there was something about the surgery that produced that effect. Doctors have no idea why this happens to many patients, but some believe that it has something to do with intestinal hormone balances.

For the first three weeks after surgery, smells drove me crazy. My sweet dog, Gambler, was banished. I couldn't stand his breath.

Some foods that patients disliked before, suddenly taste so much better. Many people report that they now enjoy spicy food in ways that they never did before. I know, because I experienced this. As an example, I was a potato chip addict. For me, any sized bag was one serving. It didn't matter if it was a medium sized bag, or a huge party-sized bag. It was one serving and I would polish it off. I could never resist potato chips. Now, I have no desire for potato chips. I have tried them on several occasions, but that is it. I'll have a chip or two and wonder what the great attraction was. Now, when I have them in our house, they actually get stale and I have to throw them away! Conversely, I stopped into a local Chinese restaurant one day and ordered a bowl of won ton soup to go. When I arrived at my office and opened the container, I discovered that they had given me hot and sour soup, not won ton. I have never liked hot and sour soup, but I had no time to return it. So I tried it. I found that I suddenly liked hot and sour soup! My tastes have changed.

At first it seemed that everything had a metallic taste. I have no idea what that was all about. Now, I look at something and it looks good. I smell the aroma and it smells wonderful. But when I taste it, something is different. I know that "something" is me. I still enjoy food, but fortunately not in the way I did before. Now I taste each bite, chew it well and savor it. I no longer eat mounds of food obsessively, because I was never satisfied and never felt full. I have made a permanent trade. I have traded food ruling my life, for a real life that is healthier and happier.

Bad Breath

Bad breath is an inevitable side effect of weight loss surgery. As your body burns fat, your mouth becomes the chimney as your body goes into a mode of ketosis. Brushing your teeth and tongue, drinking water and sucking on a sugarless mint will help. The ketosis will diminish as your weight loss slows.

Grazing

Grazing is the act of continuously eating small amounts of food throughout the entire day. This is the one way that you will be able to sabotage your surgery. Weight loss surgery is only a tool for losing weight that requires the use of a set of rules that must be followed if you want to be successful. The surgery does not produce a magic spell that allows you to continuously eat all day and still lose weight.

You might ask, "What is going on here?" "I thought my new pouch would not allow me to overeat." "I thought I would throw up if I ate too much?" What is happening is this. When you graze, you eat a small amount of food that may, or may not, fill your pouch. After a few minutes, the pouch partially empties and you fill it up again. After a few minutes, you repeat the cycle again. You are constantly moving small amounts of food through your pouch, and the total quantity of food adds up quickly. Your pouch never has a chance to empty completely to give you a sense of real hunger.

Grazing is the one way you can defeat this surgery.

If you are grazing, you are experiencing compulsive eating and will need to work through these issues with a psychologist.

Dumping

Dumping is a result of intolerance to foods that are high in sugar content and it affects approximately 70 percent of RNY surgery patients. When RNY patients eat sweets, the sugar rushes directly into the intestines without being partially digested by the gastric juices of the old stomach. In order to help break the sugar down, the body sends blood and energy to that area making the patient fell awful. They develop nausea, they may vomit, become lightheaded, dizzy, have cramps and diarrhea. These symptoms usually last about 20 to 30 minutes. This reaction is so unpleasant that dumping acts as a deterrent to eating sweets and helps with the weight loss process.

The dumping syndrome may not last forever. Most patients adjust, and are eventually able to eat some sweets after about three to six months. It is impossible to know if you will be affected by dumping or what level of sweets will trigger it. While dumping affects most people, it doesn't mean that you will never be able to eat sweets. You will probably be able to eat small amounts, but never the whole pie.

Some patients develop a mild form of dumping syndrome from eating carbohydrates. As the carbohydrates are converted to sugar, the patient feels extremely tired and sleepy. Patients, who are newly post-op, may also experience a persistent, mild nausea after eating carbohydrates. This will eventually pass.

Many patients consider dumping to be an advantageous side effect of surgery, especially if they have been sweet eaters in the past. Dumping provides them with a very strong deterrent from eating sweets and therefore, makes it easier for them to lose weight. By the time the dumping syndrome has resolved itself, the patient has learned healthier eating patterns.

Dumping can be considered an advantage. The adverse effects of eating sugar, teach you very fast to stay away from those sweets.

Although I have not totally avoided sweets, I have never personally experienced dumping. I have heard so many horror stories that I have been fearful of testing it. I have eaten a forkful or two of pie or cake or a bit of chocolate, but that's it. When I have a craving for sweets (which is now very rare), one or two bites totally satisfies me.

Not all sugars are created equal and it is sometimes difficult to identify what is sugar and what is not. Sugar is hidden everywhere. In ingredients, look for the suffix "ose." If "ose" appears at the end of an ingredient, you know it is some form of sugar. What follows is a list of sugars. Some of them can cause problems, and some usually do not. But remember, your system is unique; therefore, you need to discover what you do and do not tolerate.

**Sugars that may cause an
adverse reaction include:**

Brown Sugar	Corn Syrup
High Fructose Corn Syrup	Dextrose
Honey	Maple Syrup
Molasses	Raw Sugar
Sucrose (table sugar)	

**Simple sugars that are well tolerated
in larger amounts include:**

Fructose (fruit sugar)	Lactose (milk sugar)
Dextrin	Galactose
Glucose	Invert Sugar
Maltose	Sorbitol
Sorghum	Turbaned Sugar (Turbinado)
Xylitiol	

Remember, "no sugar added," does not mean "sugar free." Check the number of grams of sugar on the nutritional value label for the amount of sugar and determine what your particular level of tolerance is.

Taking Pills Post-Op

It is important to continue your prescribed medications post-op. But you may be concerned about taking pills that are large fearing that they might get stuck. You can try crushing your pills and putting them in something like a little bit of applesauce. Or you can buy a pill splitter to cut them in half. However, be careful if you take timed or sustained released medication. Check with your doctor or pharmacist to determine if the medication you take falls into this category. These medications are not designed to be crushed and can release medications too quickly into your system.

Timed and sustained release medications may no longer be the best choice if you have had gastric bypass surgery. These are designed to slowly break down in the stomach and intestines. Because of the change in your anatomy, they may not be absorbed correctly. Immediate release medications seem to be better suited for gastric bypass patients. Talk to your doctor about this.

Also, be sure that your primary care physician understands how rapidly you will be losing weight. Many conditions are drastically improved soon after weight loss surgery including diabetes and high blood pressure. Your physician needs to monitor your medications so that they are correct for your changing needs. A patient from my local support group was on blood pressure medication and about a month or two after surgery started complaining of dizziness and feeling faint. When her problem was isolated, her doctor discovered that her high blood pressure medication was now too strong for her, causing her blood pressure to drop too low, making her feel faint.

Most surgeons can provide you with a list of over-the-counter medications that are acceptable to take post-op. In general, any nonsteroid anti-inflammatory drug is not acceptable because they tend to cause bleeding and stomach ulcers.

The following list is a general guide to over-the-counter drugs. Be sure to check with your own surgeon to ensure that he or she agrees with these recommendations.

Medications to Avoid

Advil	Alka-Seltzer
Vanquish	Aspirin
Bufferin	Coricidin
Cortisone	Excedrin
Fiorinol	Ibuprofen
Motrin	Pepto-Bismol

Medications That Are Recommended For Colds

Benadryl	Dimetapp
Robitussin	Sudafed
Triaminics	Tylenol Cold Products

Medications That Are Usually Well Tolerated
(Try to obtain sugar free or diabetic formulas for any of these products.)

Peri-Colace	Panadol
Tylenol	Tylenol Extra Strength
Gas-X	Phazyme
Colace	Dulcolax Suppositories
Fleet Enemas	Glycerin Suppositories
Milk of Magnesia	

Dealing With Nausea

Many people have problems with nausea for their first few months post-op. Nausea can be caused by many things. Many people try to rush what their new stomachs are ready to handle. They become fearful that the way they are eating now is the way they will always eat, and push themselves to eat more, because that is what feels "normal." If you have nausea, you may want to go back to liquids for a week and then try solid food again. Take it slowly.

A lot of times, nausea is caused by your desire to eat "normally" again. "Normally" is how you got here in the first place.

Add new foods gradually so that you know what bothers you. But remember that the foods that go down well one day may cause you nausea another day. With meats, start with ground meat that is easier to chew and digest. Remember that your new pouch doesn't have the ability to digest. Shrimp and lobster were always easy for me to handle and I always ate a lot of those. Red meat is very hard to digest and most people cannot handle it until they are at least six months to a year post-op. Many people also have problems tolerating chicken because it is so dry. Dark meat is better tolerated than white meat. Try marinating meats and then cooking them in sauces until they fall apart.

Another nausea causing practice is eating too fast. I know this from first-hand experience. Slow it down unless you want to have your dinner come right back up. Remember to chew, chew, chew.

An additional cause of nausea may be the delayed function of the "Y" limb of the bowels following RNY surgery. This resolves itself over time, but is still troublesome to you if it is causing nausea.

Some people are troubled by nausea in the morning when they are newly post-op. Slowly sipping a cup of chamomile tea the first thing in the morning seems to help. Ginger pills are another natural remedy that you can try. Peppermint is a natural way to deal with nausea. Essential oil of peppermint is available at health food stores or peppermint flavoring can be purchased at grocery stores. Dilute these with water and sip them slowly. Basil leaves and basil tea are another natural remedy.

I have heard of an aromatherapy treatment that is reputed to work quite well. It sounds a little unorthodox, but if you are nauseated, you may be willing to try anything. In a small bottle mix two ounces of grapeseed oil, ten drops of peppermint oil and five drops of chamomile oil. All of these essential oils can be found in nutrition or health food stores. When you are nauseated, rub a drop or two of the oil on your stomach or if not convenient, on your wrist. Also, inhale the oils for a minute or so. The effects of the aromatherapy should be immediate.

If all of these remedies are ineffective, definitely talk to your doctor. There is no reason to endure constant nausea. There are medications that he or she can prescribe to help you.

Vomiting

Vomiting can be very common, but it can also be very serious if you are vomiting excessively. If you eat too fast and too much, chances are you will throw up. However, if you are vomiting excessively, you will probably become dangerously dehydrated. This will require you to go back into the hospital to determine what is causing your vomiting and to rehydrate you. Definitely call your surgeon as soon as possible.

Dr. Mathias Fobi, of the Center for the Surgical Treatment of Obesity in California, suggests trying a test using popcorn to determine if your vomiting is caused by an obstruction problem with the surgery or if it is caused by your eating too much or too fast or not chewing your food enough. He suggests that the patient eat popcorn and if this stays down, then there is not a physical or obstruction problem that is causing vomiting. Popcorn can only be eaten if it is chewed well and in small quantities.

As I stated earlier, I have a lot of experience with eating too fast. I almost immediately feel a sharp pain in the middle of my chest, just above my breasts. I then start to salivate (ugh). At this point, I know it is time to make my way to the bathroom and up everything comes. I am then careful not to eat or drink anything for at least an hour. My pouch always feels a little tender after a bout like this, and I try to take it easy.

Vomiting post-op is not like vomiting pre-op. Because you have no gastric juice in your pouch, you have no unpleasant taste. You are also regurgitating a very small amount so the experience is far less traumatic than what you may associate with vomiting in the past.

Endoscopy

RNY patients sometimes experience swelling of the stoma, which is the opening between the new stomach and the intestines. Sometimes this opening becomes so small that it causes vomiting when food becomes stuck. A device called an endoscope will be required to stretch the stoma to a more livable size. This very simple and painless procedure is sometimes performed in the surgeon's office. Your throat is numbed so that there is little discomfort. A tube, with a camera on the end, is put down your throat. If the opening is deemed too small, the end of the tube is inflated and the stoma is stretched. One of the medications used for this procedure is Versid, which is a medication that produces amnesia so that the patient does not remember any of the procedure.

Food Blockage

If you have had an RNY procedure, it may happen that you will get food stuck in your stoma (the opening between the pouch and the intestines). Usually, the food will dissolve by itself or will work its way through on its own.

If it is meat that is causing the blockage, one solution is to sip a cup of warm water with a pinch of dissolved meat tenderizer. It is very important that you sip very slowly because with your stoma blocked, the water will have no place to go and you will vomit.

If you have other food obstructions, one option you may have is to chew papaya tablets to aid the break up and digestion of the blockage.

A blockage can also come from fibrous vegetables. This happened to me with cooked, whole leaf spinach. The pain was terrible, and lasted for many hours. Watch out for the stalks of asparagus, broccoli, celery, etc. as well as the membranes from citrus fruits.

Lactose Intolerance

Even if you have never had problems with milk products before surgery, you may be surprised to find that you have problems now. Lactose, which is milk sugar, is absorbed through the action of an enzyme that is found in the part of the intestines that has been bypassed. Eating or drinking dairy products may now cause you nausea, cramping or gas. Since a form of sugar, mainly lactose, is present in milk, problems of dumping may occur. These conditions usually disappear within months of surgery.

Diarrhea and Constipation

Digestive problems are very common post-operatively. Your system is new and needs time to heal so that it functions properly again. Also, you are not eating the way you have done in the past. Your system is not accustomed to this and may rebel in unpleasant ways.

Diarrhea is very common in patients who have had distal bypasses. But eating certain foods that you may no longer tolerate well may also cause diarrhea. Common problem-causing foods include those high in fat and sugar, milk products and caffeine.

There are several remedies that you can try. First of all, avoid those foods containing high amounts of fat, sugar, milk and caffeine. None of them are good food choices and should be avoided, even if they did not cause you problems. Do not eat and drink at the same time. Try taking Metamucil or try the BRAT diet, which is a diet that most parents are aware of, and Pediatricians often recommend. The diet consists of eating ripe bananas, rice, applesauce (unsweetened), tea (decaffeinated) and toast (whole wheat). These are all very high in carbohydrates, so you may want to limit this diet to no more than two days.

The most effective remedy, however may be to eat yogurt or drink buttermilk. The healthy bacteria in these cultures may help your body to rid itself of the unhealthy bacteria in your digestive system that is causing the diarrhea. You may also take Lactobacillus Acidophilus, which is the same culture that is found in yogurt. It can be found in health food stores and most drug stores. If the diarrhea continues, consult with your doctor. It is important to avoid dehydration.

Constipation is another common problem. This is often the result of not drinking enough fluids, eating a diet high in animal fat, or not eating enough fiber. Foods that are high in fiber are a problem for RNY surgery patients because fiber can block the opening (stoma) between the pouch and the intestines. Also, the normal weight loss surgery diet tends to be very low in fiber. If you are eating your protein first, this leaves little room for fibrous food. Constipation can also become a problem when not eating enough food because your bowels tend to go to sleep or become semi-dormant. When in this state, they tend not to move waste products forward.

As a rule, if more than three days have passed without a bowel movement, the contents in the bowels tend to harden causing constipation. It is not necessary to have a bowel movement every day, in fact, with some people, a bowel movement every three days is normal. Avoid taking stimulant laxatives when constipated. These include Correctol, Ex Lax, Dulcolax, Senokot and Fletcher's Castoria. It is very easy for your body to become dependent upon them and you may reach a point where you cannot have a bowel movement without taking a stimulant laxative. Stimulant laxatives should never be taken more than twice a week. However, a stool softener may be used anytime it is needed. These include Colace, Dialose and Surfak. Your body does not become dependent upon these, and they may bring you relief. Bulk-forming laxatives are considered the safest. These are taken with water and cause water to be absorbed in the colon making the stool softer. These include products such as FiberCon, Metamucil, and Citrucel.

Avoid taking stimulant laxatives. Your
body can become dependent upon them.

If constipation lasts for more than three weeks, talk to your doctor. As a last resort, there is a prescription medication called MiraLax that can be very helpful.

28
Exercise That New Body

Check with your doctor concerning when you are able to start exercising. Most will say to start walking immediately. Walking is very important in the healing process and especially important to help prevent blood clots. For more strenuous exercising, you should probably wait two or three weeks. Your doctor will be the best judge.

Exercise is especially important following weight loss surgery because you will be losing weight so rapidly. When your body realizes how rapidly your weight is decreasing, it goes into a panic state and tries to hold onto the stores of fat to prevent starvation. When this happens, the body will burn muscle mass and hold onto stored fat, which is just what you do not want your body to do. To combat this, it is important to regularly exercise vigorously so that your metabolism increases and your body burns fat and not muscle mass.

The reality is, few people enjoy exercising. But you've got to do it!

If you are like me, you probably did not do much exercising before surgery. My back was so bad that it was difficult enough to deal with everyday living much less an exercise program. I started out slowly. I bought a recumbent exercise bicycle with a full seat that tilts back, which was very easy on my back. When I felt that I wanted to add something else, I added lifting hand weights while I pedaled. After a few months, I started going to a gym. While I am still not an enthusiastic exerciser, I do understand its importance, so I try to keep exercise as a part of my life.

Pick an exercise to do that you enjoy. If you hate walking, then bicycle or skate, use a stair stepper, do water aerobics, sweat to the oldies, play golf or tennis. Make what you do enjoyable and convenient, or you won't do it. If you decide to take an aerobics class, try to have a friend do it with you. Listen to music or a book on tape while exercising. Read or watch TV while on exercise machines.

Start out slowly. You will be walking laps around the nurses' station at the hospital and you will need to continue moving when you get home. During the first six weeks following surgery, walking is the best form of exercise. You will be very tired and not able to do much initially. You have gone through major surgery, and your body is directing all of its energy to healing. I started exercising my first week. I did all of five minutes on the treadmill everyday. I then worked that up to fifteen minutes. I took it easy so I wouldn't hurt myself, but not so easy that I was really babying myself.

Life style changes can also affect your level of fitness. Start to take the stairs instead of the elevator. Try parking at the far end of the parking lot rather than waiting for a spot nearby to open up. Get up, stretch and walk around as frequently as possible when you are working in your office. Carry groceries, rake leaves, mow the lawn, and do gardening. In general, try to be as active as you can. If you mold your daily activity to be exercise intensive, you will be constantly moving to a higher level of physical fitness.

There are some excellent exercise videos for larger people, people who are totally out of shape, and people who have bad knees or backs. Appendix D contains some titles that you might want to look into getting. Please remember to get approval from your doctor before starting any exercise program.

Aerobic Exercise

Aerobic exercise, which means, "exercise with oxygen," requires continuous motion. This type of exercise is very important to increase your heart rate and your metabolism so that you will burn more body fat.

Types of aerobic exercise include using a stair stepper, walking rapidly on a treadmill (especially if it is inclined), and walking outside in uneven terrain. Elliptical machines provide low-impact exercise, which is excellent for those having joint and back problems. Bicycling, jogging, aerobic dancing and swimming are other forms of aerobic exercise. For those who have difficulty moving, water aerobics provides the buoyancy that supports you and allows you to move and exercise.

Target Heart Rate

When doing aerobic exercising, determine what your target heart rate is. To compute this number, subtract your age from 220. Because you want your target heart rate to be between 60 percent and 75 percent for effective fat burning, multiply this number times .6 to .75 depending upon your endurance. For example, if you are 35 years old and are just starting aerobic exercising, you would subtract 35 from 220, which would equal 185. You would then multiply 185 times .6 (or up to .75), which would equal 111. This is the number of beats per minute that you want your heart to beat during an aerobic exercise. To count the beats per minute, find your pulse on the inside of your wrist or on your neck about two inches down from your ear. Another way to find your pulse on your neck is to put your index and middle fingers on your Adam's apple and move your fingers straight back until you feel your pulse. Once you have your pulse, count your heartbeat for 15 seconds and multiply the number times 4. This will give you your heart rate.

Another way to determine your heart rate is to use a device that continuously reads your heart rate. Some aerobic machines have them. The heart rate monitor is built into the handlebar of the machine, or there is a separate clip that attaches to your finger. Another type is a monitor that you wear around your midriff that also uses a monitor that looks like a watch that you wear around your wrist. These are sold in most sporting goods stores and are very convenient and accurate to use.

Try to continue the intensity so that you are maintaining your target heart rate. As you do more exercising, you will have to increase the intensity as your heart becomes more efficient. The object is to maintain that fat burning rate for at least 20 consecutive minutes. Adding additional time for warm up and cool down will probably mean that you will have to exercise continuously for at least 30 minutes. Do this at least three times per week. For weight loss, it is recommended that 1,000 calories per week be burned as a result of exercise. There are many charts and books available that will indicate the number of calories that are burned during a particular activity for your current weight. Various exercise machines will also provide you with this number as you are exercising.

For weight loss, it is recommended that 1,000 calories per week be burned as a result of exercise.

If the only way that you can exercise is in short bursts of 10-minute intervals, then go with that. The point is that you must exercise. If short bursts are all that you can manage, then that is better than not exercising at all. It is much better to exercise in a way that will ensure that you will continue on a regular schedule, rather than not exercising at all because you don't have the time, the endurance, or the desire to exercise for longer stretches of time.

Anaerobic Exercise

Anaerobic exercise works to improve your overall physical condition, but does not improve your heart and lungs. A typical anaerobic exercise would be weight lifting. Although weight lifting will not burn as many calories as jogging, for instance, it will build your muscles. You want to decrease fat in your body and increase your muscle mass. One pound of muscle burns about 35 calories per day, so the more muscle mass you have, the more calories you will burn.

The Good News and the Bad News About Exercising

Here's the good news first. As you exercise, you will lose more weight because you are burning calories and increasing your metabolism. This is especially important to keep your weight from plateauing excessively. So in one sense the more you exercise, the more weight you will lose. Exercise is also important to help maintain muscle tone as you are losing.

Now, here is the bad news. Muscle mass weighs more than body fat. So when you exercise, you are building muscle that adds to your total body weight, but at the same time you are burning fat, which decreases your weight. This means that you may experience a slowing of your weight loss as you are building muscle. But the more muscle you have, the more calories you burn. This is a trade-off that is definitely worth it. At some point, your body will adapt to the increased exercise and you will continue to lose weight at an increased rate.

Many people get discouraged when the muscle building aspect hits them and they stop losing weight. Don't let this dissuade you from exercising regularly. Exercise is a vital part of the success of this surgery. As long as you continue to follow the rules of good eating and follow a good daily exercise program, you will reach your goal.

Weight Training

Lifting hand weights is an excellent way to build up your muscles. One of your goals throughout your weight loss journey should be to increase your muscle mass. Because of the rapid weight decline experienced by weight loss surgery patients, the body has a tendency to feed off of muscle tissue rather than body fat. This is because the body goes into a preservation response and tends to hold onto its fat reserves. Therefore, any activity that deals with increasing muscle strength deserves our attention. The average woman who strength trains for eight weeks gains 1.75 pounds of muscle and loses 3.5 pounds of fat.

You can start with weights as light as 1-pound, and increase them as you gain strength. This can be especially important because as you lose weight, your muscles will be doing less work and will burn fewer calories. You want this to be the other way around. As you lose fat weight, you need to build your muscles so they will burn more fat energy.

Weight lifting is important for toning muscles and maintaining bone density.

A typical routine includes a set of six to eight exercises emphasizing the major muscle groups. Each exercise should be repeated 12 to 15 times, resting about 1 minute between sets. The same exercises should not be done every day. It is advisable to do a routine for the upper body on day 1 followed by a routine for the lower body on day 2. Alternating is important to allow the muscles to repair. A warm-up prior to starting each strength training session should be performed to raise body temperature and to get joints and muscles ready for the workout. There are some excellent books on the market that will guide you through routines.

Women should not be concerned about building up an excessive amount of muscle bulk. What you should strive for is a firm appearance to your body and not the "Ms. / Mr. America" look. Testosterone is the hormone responsible for muscle growth and women have 10 to 20 times less testosterone in their bodies than men. If you are able to maintain a firm body, you will have developed a good muscle tone that should significantly help in your weight loss efforts.

Strength training is also an excellent way to combat depression. A Harvard study found that ten weeks of strength training reduced clinical depression better than counseling did.

Additionally, strength training is an excellent way to combat loss of bone density. Wescott Research found that strength training could increase spinal bone density by 13 percent. This is an excellent way to help prevent osteoporosis.

The Body-For-Life Program

The Body-for-Life Program is a popular regimen that combines strength training three days per week and aerobic training three days per week. This is combined with a nutrition plan of six small meals a day. The strength training portion requires you to alternate upper and lower body workouts on Mondays, Wednesdays and Fridays. Aerobic exercises are done for 20 minutes on Tuesdays, Thursdays and Saturdays. Options for aerobic exercises include stationary bicycling, stair stepping, cross-country skiing, swimming, running or treadmill workouts. Each of the small meals includes a portion of protein and a portion of carbohydrate. The author of the program and best selling book, Bill Phillips, offers a challenge in which anyone may enter and win prizes based upon your improvement over a 12-week period. Many people swear by the program. See **http://www.bodyforlife.com** for details on the challenge.

29
How To Ensure Your Success

I hear so many people saying that when they hit their first plateau, they know they are going to be the one person in the world that will fail to lose weight after having weight loss surgery. Well, inevitably they start to lose weight again and breathe a sigh of relief. So when that first plateau hits, and that same thought in turn hits you, remember these rules for success. These are the rules discussed in my surgeon's support group. Follow these rules and you absolutely will not fail. Read these rules often. They are much easier to follow after your surgery when you have a small pouch to help control your hunger.

> *You will succeed if you eat protein first at any meal, drink water, exercise, and don't graze.*

Rules For Success To Loose Weight

1) **Eat Protein First**- Concentrate on your protein at each and every meal. After you have eaten your portion of protein, if there is any room left, then eat carbohydrates. The more carbohydrates you eat, the hungrier you will feel and the more you will crave them. Check with your own surgeon about eating a high protein diet. It will help tremendously with weight loss, but if you have any liver problems, it might not be a good idea for you. Let your surgeon be the judge

2) **Drink Water**- Be sure to drink at least 64 ounces of water, or non-carbonated, caffeine free liquid per day. Do not drink carbonated beverages.

3) **Exercise**- Exercise at least three days per week.

4) **No Grazing**- Do not snack. This is the one way that you can sabotage your surgery. If you are truly hungry between meals, eat a small bite of protein.

The Rules For Success Long-Term

A study was done observing characteristics of gastric bypass patients who have remained successful, long-term. This study, done by Ms. Colleen Cook and Dr. Charles Edwards, was subsequently published in the September 1999 issue of Obesity Surgery. These are their observations. There is an old saying that says "to be successful, you need to do what successful people do." If you use these observations as your own guideline, you will surely have significant results from your surgery.

Eating - Those who were successful, long-term, ate three meals and two snacks per day, which included three servings of protein, three servings of vegetables and one serving of fruit, two servings of carbohydrates and two servings of sweets. Remember that this is food that they ate after they had attained their goal weight, not what they ate as they were losing.

Drinking – Successful patients averaged 40 to 64 ounces of water per day and did not drink carbonated beverages. Only 26 percent drank alcoholic beverages and less than half drank juice or sweetened beverages.

Vitamins and Supplements - Successful patients took multiple vitamins, calcium and iron, if needed, on a daily basis.

Sleeping - Successful patients averaged seven hours of sleep per night and 3/4 of them rated their energy level as average or high.

Exercising - Those that were successful, exercised 4 times per week for 40 minutes. They credit the exercise to their ability to maintain their weight.

Personal Responsibility - Successful patients consider themselves personally responsible for their success. They believe that their success is up to them and see their surgery as a tool that they used to attain their healthy weight and maintain it. Nearly 70 percent weigh themselves at least weekly so that they can monitor their weight control.

30
Surgery Is Only A Tool

There is nothing magical about losing weight after weight loss surgery. Ninety seven percent of patients are successful as opposed to only five percent who diet. Remember that "successful" is defined as losing 50 percent of your excess weight. But if you want to reach your goal weight, you will have to apply good sense. There are rules for success, as well as ways that you can sabotage your surgery. It will still be necessary to make wise food choices and exercise some control, but this is so much easier to do post-op. You will not be able to go back to your previous way of eating and some people have a difficult time with that adjustment. You will need to make lifestyle changes. And if you eat for reasons other than hunger, you will need to have some counseling to address those issues. But, and I can't stress this enough, it is so worth the effort. When I think of how far I have come, I can't believe it. Remember that I had the same cycle of yo-yo dieting that you had. I had the same failure after failure as you. With dieting, I had the same initial success, followed by a regain of all the weight, plus more, that you had. By using weight loss surgery as a tool, I did it, and it wasn't that hard. You can too!

Weight loss surgery is a tool. How successful you are depends upon how well you use that tool.

Long term this is what you can expect. The Mayo Clinic did a study of RNY patients that were three years post-op and found the following:

- 93 percent considered themselves satisfied and improved
- 84 percent reported that they felt the same feeling of being satisfied after eating as they did soon after their surgery

> 82 percent reported an overall decrease in appetite, and all were able to eat regular food

This was three years after surgery!

Of the foods that were not well tolerated:
> 23 percent had problems with milk
> 14 percent had problems with steak
> 10 percent had problems with hamburger

Although 22 percent reported having diarrhea once or more times per week, symptoms of heartburn, vomiting and constipation were very rare.

31
Support Groups

Support can make a tremendous difference to your success. You might be fortunate enough to meet someone who is going through the surgery at the same time as you are. When you are in the hospital, be sure to ask the nurses to point out other weight loss surgery patients to you so that you can exchange phone numbers. When you are visiting your surgeon for pre-op and post-op consultations, strike up conversations with others in the waiting room. Again, exchange phone numbers and keep in touch. It helps to talk with someone when you are going through a plateau or are having other minor problems.

Your Surgeon's Support Group

Hopefully, your surgeon has a support group that meets on a regular basis. It is so important to take advantage of these. If one does not exist in your area, suggest to your surgeon that he or she start one. My surgeon, Dr. Philip Schauer, has a meeting the first Wednesday of every month from 7 to 9 PM. He and his staff are always there to present the evening's program and to answer any questions. We are particularly fortunate that three of Dr Schauer's staff are RNY patients themselves, and can answer questions from both a medical and personal level. Some meetings are informal question and answer sessions, while others are more structured with a special speaker. Topics have included plastic surgery, psychological issues, behavior modification, exercise, nutrition, and many others. Prior to the meeting, many of us meet to chat and compare notes. I know I always have a core group of people to call upon if I ever need help. I never rely on these people for medical advice. I utilize Dr. Schauer and his staff for that. But I have my weight loss surgery "buddies" there for much needed support.

On-line Support Groups

One of the best sources of support is the Internet. By going to **http://groups.yahoo.com** you can join a number of bulletin boards that cater specifically to patients of weight loss surgery. The mother of all weight loss surgery support groups is OSSG (Obesity Surgery Support Group) with currently more than 5,000 members. You can email questions to the group and receive dozens of public and private replies or you can just "lurk" and find out information gradually. When you sign up to be on the list, you can choose to have your email sent in digest form (one email with many messages) or an individual email for every message. There are at least 50 messages generated everyday, so it is helpful to set your mode to digest. The moderators will collect about 25 messages and send them out in one digest email. Topics discussed vary, but are always on the subject of weight loss surgery. This is not the place to get medical advice however; it is a place to get support from people with experience.

> *On-line support groups are wonderful but do not rely on them for medical advice. That is your surgeon's role.*

There are many variations on the OSSG theme. In addition to the main forum, there are regional OSSG forums for people living in a particular area. There is an OSSG-Graduate group for those who are 1-year or more post-op. You can join this group earlier, but you cannot post unless you are at least one year out. There is an OSSG for recipes, for insurance problems, for those interested in exercise, for those going through weight loss surgery with no family support, etc. Each list maintains an archive so that you can read past messages and search by topic.

Angel

An angel is someone who checks on you while you are in the hospital and reports back to your support group on your condition. You can build very close ties within these groups and many will know when your surgery is scheduled, and will want to follow your progress. But it will take quite a few days before you feel up to going onto the Internet yourself, so your angel is there to let everyone know how you are doing. If no one volunteers to be your angel, don't be afraid to post a message asking if anyone would like to take on that task. You will probably have many people willing to do this.

My angel was particularly helpful when I was in the hospital. I had a minor complication and asked my angel to post a question to OSSG regarding whether anyone else experienced the same problem. I was not looking for medical advice because I was in the hospital and getting excellent medical care. I just wanted to connect with someone who had gone through what I had. It made me feel much less vulnerable and hopeful that everything would be all right.

32
Psychological And Emotional Issues

As your body changes so dramatically, you will be mentally changing. These changes can be very disturbing. Many morbidly obese people have used their size to avoid or hide from life. Fat can serve as a buffer. It can insulate you from the world, providing protection from commitment, attention, and unwanted sexual advances. Losing that buffer can leave you feeling very vulnerable. If you are having trouble dealing with all the emotional issues that you may be facing as you are losing huge amounts of weight, I highly recommend that you seek professional counseling. This will help your transition go more smoothly and will better insure that you will be more successful in your weight loss journey.

Depression

So you have gone through this surgery. You have waited months for it, perhaps fought your insurance company to have it. It is what you thought you wanted. But being thinner does not solve all of your problems. You are still the same person inside. Your family members have not changed. Being thinner does not make your life perfect. It does help many things, and makes them better, such as your health problems. But it does not solve psychological problems.

> *You encounter so many changes in your weight loss surgery journey. A good counselor can help you work your way through these changes.*

Depression, following weight loss surgery, is very common for a variety of factors. First of all, for women, estrogen is running rampant through your body. As body fat is burned to produce energy, the estrogen that is stored in those fat cells is released into the blood stream, causing a hormonal surge. It is like having a very bad case of PMS. Another cause of depression is the anesthesia from your surgery. As the anesthesia leaves your system, sometimes taking up to two weeks, it is very common to experience some level of depression. And if you have been an emotional eater before surgery, you no longer have that outlet. You are at home recovering from surgery, probably watching a lot of television, and being bombarded with food commercials. You cannot eat any of the food that you see on television, as you are limited to liquids or pureed foods. Of course you are depressed!

Many patients experience what Drs. Selinkoff, Pilcher and Reiss of San Antonio, Texas refer to as "hibernation syndrome." Within two to four weeks after surgery, the body realizes that it will not be getting the nourishment that it is used to receiving and reacts to that. You feel extremely tired, lethargic, and often depressed. Your body just wants to stay immobile until the old food supply returns. This period comes at a time when you are just starting to recover from the traumatic effects of the surgery. The pain is gone and energy was just starting to return. And then the hibernation syndrome hits.

The best way to deal with the hybernation syndrome is to recognize the symptoms and know that you are normal. Then start to exercise so that your body becomes accustomed to using your own body fat as a source of fuel. As soon as your body figures out that it has ample sources of fuel stored inside, and does not have to be constantly fed, the syndrome will end. It may take as long as two weeks for this to happen.

Spousal Jealousy

It is possible that your spouse may have a difficult time dealing with your new physical identity. Not only has your body changed, but your personality may also have changed as you gain new self-confidence and self-esteem. This is a new you that your spouse may have never seen before. It is natural for your spouse to feel insecure. This jealousy might show itself in different ways. Your spouse might become overly possessive and smothering or may become distant, fearing what may seem like an inevitable end. If you see evidence of problems developing, get to a marriage counselor!

Divorce Rate

The divorce rate for couples following weight loss surgery is relatively high. This surgery can make good marriages better and bad marriages worse. Many morbidly obese women marry believing that their choice is the best that they can get or the best that they deserve. These women hate themselves and believe that no one could possibly love them. They settle gratefully for a negative relationship and some actually endure mental or verbal abuse. When they start to lose weight, become more attractive, and gain self-esteem, they question whether they need to continue in an unhappy marriage.

Dealing With New Attention

Our society places such an importance on physical appearance, especially for women. And as morbidly obese women, we have become accustomed to being ignored by most of the opposite sex. We become non-people or invisible "masses." In some cases, that was an objective. Excess weight can be used as a buffer to ward off unwanted attention. If, for whatever reason, we feel we are unworthy of attention, one way to deflect attention is through obesity. It can be used as a shield, or as an excuse for many of the failures and disappointments in our lives. As we lose weight, we become more vulnerable. We no longer have an excuse for not facing the world. This can sometimes be a very frightening state. It is best to seek counseling in these situations.

As we start to lose weight, we discover that we are receiving new attention. Members of the opposite sex are flirting with us, sometimes for the first times in our lives. For those of us who have been obese forever, we are adolescents when it comes to dealing with flirting. We are totally out of our depths. We have no experience to know when someone is flirting innocently and when someone is serious. Before acting on flirting, stop, take a breath, and consider what you may have to win or lose, the benefits and the consequences.

> *We have no experience to know when someone is flirting innocently and when someone is serious.*

Friends

Losing a great deal of weight can disrupt relationships. You are changing every day, and you may find that your friends are unwilling or unable to change in the relationship along with you. Your friends may very well be feeling jealousy or resentment. You may be accustomed to a certain routine with your friends. If a lot of your activities revolved around eating, it could put distance between you and your friends when you just do not enjoy going out to eat as much as you used to.

Initially, you will be restricted in what you can eat and certainly in the amount. I know it was a real turn-off for me to sit in a restaurant and see the mountains of food that people ate. Although I ate huge amounts of food prior to my surgery, I looked at food in a different way and was amazed at how much people would consume. I also wanted to be up and doing things other than sitting at a table stuffing my mouth with food. I had a new level of energy that I hadn't had in 20 years. I wanted to golf, bicycle, walk around the mall, move! I didn't want to be inactive anymore.

If you are feeling some of this, your friends may not understand. They may say that you have changed and are not the same person anymore. And they will be absolutely correct! Hopefully, they will be happy for you and stay close. Friends are wonderful, and you should make every effort to hold onto them, if you can. But if you can't, don't feel guilty. Know in your mind that you have taken steps to create a better and healthier life for yourself and tried to make the friendship work. At some point, you may sadly need to realize that the friendship was an important chapter in your life, and one that you will always cherish, but it is time to move on.

When Am I Going To Wake Up Thin?

Not long after my surgery, I had a difficult time when I realized that I was not going to become thin overnight. I felt that when I told people that I had weight loss surgery, they would look at me and correctly assess that I was still fat! I would always ask myself, "If I had the surgery, why wasn't I thin?" And despite that I knew that this surgery is only a "tool," the idea of yet again having to watch carefully what I ate, was discouraging. I wanted to be thin right now. I had waited long enough to have the surgery; waited for appointments, waited to be approved by my insurance company, and waited for an available surgery date. Why couldn't I be thin right now? And how long would this process take?

Well I finally did calm down, as most patients do, and got into a routine with my life. And one wonderful day, I did wake up thin! I'll never forget the morning that I looked into my bathroom mirror and came face to face with my true body size. I finally found the thin person that was hiding inside me.

I looked in the mirror and said, "There you are. I finally found you. I knew there was a thin person hiding in there."

Body Image

We all have a sense of our bodies and how we relate to others and our environment. But when our bodies go through such a rapid and drastic change, we tend to lose a sense of ourselves and can actually undergo an identity crisis. Patients report that when they pass someone, they still give people a wide berth as if their bodies are still the same large size. They tend to go through a turnstile sideways even though it is no longer necessary. And catching their reflection in a glass can be very disconcerting. They don't recognize themselves. It is like they are walking around in someone else's body. It takes some getting used to.

Shopping For Clothes

Shopping for new clothes can be equally disturbing. We have been waiting for so long to fit into these new slim clothes and we don't know where to go to get them. We are accustomed to going to Lane Bryant or another "plus-size" store and picking out what fits and not really thinking about it. Now you can walk in and out of stores and be so frustrated trying to find just where you "fit in." In what department in what store do you shop? You have to decide what brands you now like, and what is "you." You have to establish a new identity. It can be fun trying on those clothes that you just can't believe fit you now. And it can be a bit scary. But you do find your way, and eventually shopping will be enjoyable as you find yourself sobbing with joy in the dressing room, when you slip on a size you haven't worn in years. You just need to give yourself time.

It is a great feeling when you walk into a regular size store, and realize that the saleslady knows, from the beginning, that you are shopping for yourself and not for some slim friend or relative. You actually belong in that store because you need slim clothes for yourself.

You will definitely need to buy some clothes along the way. You will look and feel much better if you aren't wearing baggy clothes. You don't have to spend a tremendous amount of money, but do adapt your wardrobe to your diminishing size. Many people shop in second-hand shops or shop on eBay.com. This is a great way to save some money on a temporary wardrobe. Also, many support groups have clothing exchanges so that at least you know that your clothes are going to a good home and you can pick out some items for yourself.

If you are like me, you have a wide range of sizes in your closet. I had sizes from 24/26 down to size 12. And I went through them all as I lost weight. I was sure that size 14 was the size I would end up wearing, so I started to buy clothes in that size. Well, the size 14 clothes got too big and I ended up having more sizes on the way down. I would have thought that I gave up those multiple sizes when I lost weight. I still had multiple sizes, but instead of outgrowing them because they were too small, I was outgrowing them because they were too big. Buy some clothes that fit, but don't buy an extensive wardrobe until your weight truly stabilizes.

One of the things that I have always been fearful of in the past was throwing away old clothing as I got smaller. I had become so accustomed to regaining weight after dieting, that I felt it was hardly worth the effort of throwing the clothes away because I knew they would fit again. I would regain the weight as I had always done, and the pounds would probably bring along some friends. This time was different. I knew when I lost the weight this time that it was gone forever and I would never see those old sizes again. So as I got smaller, I found it amazingly easy to pitch those old sizes.

It will never come back. Every pound is gone forever. Finally, I won!
Linnann

If you have suits in sizes that have become too big for you, you may want to consider donating them to Dress For Success. Dress For Success is a non-profit organization that was founded in 1996. The organization is in 60 cities in 4 countries and has helped over 60,000 low-income women dress professionally for the workforce. For each woman that they help, they give one suit for an interview. When she gets a job, she receives a second suit for work. The organization takes donations of skirt and pant suits with good matching blouses. They also accept blazers, jackets, and new or nearly new dress shoes. They are particularly in need of larger sizes. They do ask that the clothing be in good and clean condition. For more information, their website is **http://www.dressforsuccess.org**.

33
Post-Op and
Longer Term Considerations

Window of Opportunity

There is a time period of 12 to 18 months, immediately following your surgery, during which you have the greatest opportunity to lose weight. This is called your "window of opportunity." Immediately following surgery, you cannot eat and will be on a liquid diet until your new pouch heals. As you slowly transition into solid food you will be eating extremely small amounts. Not only will you have a very small stomach that holds about one ounce of food, your new stomach will also be swollen from the surgery. You will experience fullness and satiety from very little food. Most people find that there are many days when they actually forget to eat! It is important to take advantage of this time, before your hunger returns. Your new stomach will stretch a bit so that you will eventually be able to eat from four to eight ounces of food, but that will take a number of months. It is very important to learn new eating habits during this time period. These lessons will help you to maintain your weight in the months to come.

Take every advantage of the first 12 months to lose as much weight as you can. It will never be this easy again.

When Will I Stop Losing Weight?

People commonly asked me how I would stop losing weight. This was apparently a great concern when every time they would see me, I would be smaller. I suppose they imagined that one day I would just blow away. As you get smaller, your body expends less energy moving. This means that your calorie requirements are less. Because of this, your weight loss will slow and eventually stop or stabilize as you approach your ideal weight. You are just not burning the calories that you burned when your body was larger.

Pregnancy

For some women, one of the reasons for having weight loss surgery is their inability to conceive. Estrogen is stored in fat cells and as women gain fat cells it affects their fertility. As they begin to lose weight and lose fat cells, pre-menopausal women experience a new-found fertility. Added to this possibility of pregnancy, is a more active sex life as you become more physically attractive and begin to feel better about yourself. Women, who have not had a period in years, suddenly find that they have begun again.

Eighty percent of patients having weight loss surgery are women in their childbearing years. It is very important to remember to not become pregnant within the first year following surgery, to give your body time to adjust. In the beginning months following surgery, it is difficult to get in a sufficient amount of nutrition to satisfy all your own bodily needs and nearly impossible to supply the nutritional needs of a growing fetus. During the first year after surgery, pregnancy is considered to be high risk and the possibility of a miscarriage is increased by 90 percent.

It is very important to not become pregnant within the first year following surgery. After that, you should be "good to go!"

Another factor that creates a high-risk pregnancy is that morbidly obese women commonly have co-morbidities such as high blood pressure and diabetes that puts increased stress on the body. The addition of a pregnancy could endanger the health of the mother.

Therefore, if you are at all sexually active, it is very important to use birth control during the first year after surgery. You may very well have a healthy baby, but the risk is not worth it. Wait the year, for your own sake as well as for the sake of your baby.

However, once you have received an approval from your surgeon or obstetrician to become pregnant, you should have a very normal pregnancy. In the August 1998 issue of <u>Obesity Surgery</u>, Dr. Wittgrove et al reported on a study conducted following 41 of their own gastric bypass patients who had become pregnant. Their pregnancies were normal and their deliveries were without complications.

Incision Scar

If you have had an open procedure, you may experience itching as the incision line heals. Here is a remedy that you may want to try to promote healing, reduce scaring and reduce itching. Once your incision has completely closed, apply 10,000 IU vitamin E oil in the following manner. Massage the oil into the incision area and the surrounding area. Put a piece of clear plastic wrap over the area. Place a warm, damp towel over the plastic wrap. Place a dry towel over the warm damp towel. Put a heating pad over this with the setting on medium. Lie back and relax. Do this for 20 minutes, 2 times per day for 2 weeks. This helps the incision line to heal flat with less scaring.

Sleeping Problems

Some people report difficulty sleeping. This is not from pain, but they seem to wake up in the middle of the night and be unable to get back to sleep. This may be caused by low blood sugar. Try eating some protein just before going to bed, or have some protein at your bedside, such as nuts. Hopefully this will help.

Feeling Cold

About half of those who have had weight loss surgery complain that they are always cold. There seems to be no definitive reason for this. If you do experience this, some have said that increasing their protein level has helped.

Hair Loss

There is good news and bad news. The bad news is that one third of the people who have weight loss surgery lose up to one half of their hair. It actually comes out in handfuls. The hair loss usually starts around the third or fourth month. It seems to be caused by the body's reaction to the trauma of surgery.

The bad news continues. There doesn't seem to be much you can do about it. Keeping up your protein, taking zinc pills and biotin may help a little, but not enough to really make much of a difference for most patients. Minoxidil products may limit how much you will lose, but if your body reacts this way, the use of these products and medication will not help.

I have never known anyone who has lost all of his or her hair; so don't think that this surgery will result in your looking like a cue ball! Getting your hair cut in a shorter style makes it look fuller, so that is an option. Not everyone experiences hair loss. But if it is you, it can be very traumatic while you are going through it. I was one of the lucky ones. I didn't experience any hair loss at all.

Hair loss doesn't happen to everyone. But if it happens to you, it can be traumatic. Just remember that it all grows back!

Now, here is the good news. It comes back because the hair loss is only temporary. Around the fifth or sixth month, it starts to grow back in. Soon you have your normal head of hair back. And you can then breathe a sigh of relief!

Back Pain

It is common for people who have never had back pain to now have it after they have lost a large amount of weight. As your body changes, your center of gravity changes and your muscles and joints aren't used to this. Working with a physical therapist or a chiropractor helps. Also, people complain of tailbone pain. They are accustomed to a large cushion of fat around their tailbone. When they lose the weight, they feel like they are sitting directly on their tailbone. A rubber ring will help until your body adjusts.

Bone Density

One of the few physical advantages that heavy people have is bone density. Because of the excess weight, bones respond by growing strong enough to provide support. Bone mass is not static. It is vibrant tissue that responds to our weight, what we eat, and what we do. As we lose weight, bone density becomes less, because it does not have to provide as much support. Preserving bone density should become a major concern to us as our bones become naturally thinner as we lose weight.

There are many ways to preserve bone density. One very effective way to preserve and increase your bone density is to exercise with weights. As you do weight bearing exercises such as weight lifting, you are adding stress and strain to your bones. This stress causes your bones to respond in a manner that is similar to bones in an overweight person, by stimulating the formation of new bone. A weight bearing exercise program can increase bone mass by as much as five to ten percent. Walking and jogging can maintain bone density, but if you are looking to increase it, you must participate in a program of weight lifting at least two times per week.

Diet is also important to maintain bone density. A high protein diet, which most weight loss surgery patients eat, is actually detrimental to bone density. Bones store the majority of calcium, phosphorus and magnesium in our body. When these minerals are low in our blood stream, the body breaks down bone to replace them. When we eat protein, the body needs calcium to neutralize the acidic protein products that have been broken down. Since the majority of calcium resides in our bones, the body breaks down bones to free up this calcium. This is one reason why calcium supplements are so important to take. A daily regimen of 1,000 to 1,500 mg of calcium will help to give your bones additional strength. See the section on calcium in Chapter 25, for the correct form of calcium to take.

Hormones such as estrogen also build bone density. This is important especially if you are a post-menopausal woman. Hormone replacement therapy however, should be discussed with your physician or gynecologist to consider all of the side effects. For those who choose not to take hormone therapy, or for anyone concerned about bone density, Ipriflavone can be used. Ipriflavone is a new synthetic product that, according to studies, prevents bone mineral loss. It works to inhibit bone breakdown and facilitates bone building. The dosage in most of the studies was 600 mg per day in 3 divided doses.

Follow up

It is very important to comply with your surgeon's follow-up program, which is normally referred to as "aftercare." Aftercare usually involves a visit with your surgeon at the one-month, three-month, six-month and twelve-month anniversaries of your surgery. During the early visits you will inevitable have many questions that deal with adjusting to your new eating habits. Some foods will trouble you and you will be able to address this. Your surgeon will also have the opportunity to ensure that you completely understand what will help you to be totally successful with this surgery, how to stay healthy, and how best to utilize this wonderful tool. During many of these appointments, your blood levels will probably be checked to determine any early deficiencies. Check with your surgeon's staff to determine if you should fast for any of these appointments.

Aftercare can ensure your success. Your surgeon can monitor your health to be sure that you are staying on track.

The second year, visits are every six months to a year. During these visits your weight will be monitored and the staff can address any problems that you might be having dealing with a now slightly larger pouch and the ability to eat almost anything. After the second year, an annual visit is required. Patients who are successful, commit to these follow-up sessions.

Aftercare can ensure your success. Your surgeon can monitor your health to be sure that you are staying on track.

34
Plastic Surgery

Plastic surgery is often required or desired after patients have lost a large amount of weight. Often this surgery is reconstructive more than cosmetic. Depending upon your age, type of skin, how much weight you have lost, and how long you have been overweight, you may still be left with excess skin that will just not go away, regardless of how much weight you lose and how much you exercise. This skin can be more than a nuisance. It can cause significant health problems such as back strain or pain, skin rashes and infections, and sexual dysfunctions. Excess folds of skin can cause difficulty fitting into clothes, problems with personal hygiene, difficulty walking and the possibility of psychological problems from the feelings of disfigurement.

You won't want to have plastic surgery until you lose all your excess weight and your weight stabilizes.

Because of these medical problems, abdominoplasties, breast reductions and other plastic surgery procedures are often covered by insurance. In order for insurance companies to pay for plastic surgeries, they must determine that they are medically necessary and not cosmetic. Proof of medical necessity must be established by having the surgeon document the condition in the patient's medical history. In some cases, insurance companies will require photographs to substantiate the insurance claim.

The following definition of cosmetic and reconstructive surgery was adopted by the American Medical Association, June 1989:
"Cosmetic Surgery is performed to reshape normal structures of the body in order to improve the patient's appearance and self esteem. Reconstructive surgery is performed on abnor-

mal structures of the body, caused by congenital defects, developmental abnormalities, trauma, infection, tumors, or disease. It is generally performed to improve function but may also be done to approximate a normal appearance."

Panniculectomy and Abdominoplasty

The most common problem area is the large apron of excess skin in the abdominal area known as the "panniculus." If this area of excess skin does not shrink, the only way to deal with it is to surgically remove it. The removal of this excess skin is called a panniculectomy. An abdominoplasty involves tightening the abdominal wall and then removing usually about six to twelve pounds of excess skin and tissue. Because of medical problems that can develop, panniculectomies and abdominoplasties are often covered by insurance.

According to the American Society of Plastic Surgeons, an excess of ten pounds of tissue in the abdominal area adds 100 pounds of strain on the disks of the lower back by exaggerating the normal "S" curve of the spine.

Breast Reconstruction

Many women require reconstructive breast surgery. These procedures are sometimes covered by insurance if they are considered medically necessary because of back pain, neck and shoulder pain, skin rash and infection.

Upper Arms

Excess skin in the upper arms, often known as "batwings" is another problem area. Because this is not an area that causes medical problems, it is rarely covered by insurance.

Thighs

Excess skin in the thigh area is also problematic. Liposuction can sometimes be effective. Excess skin can be surgically removed, but the long incision can sometimes heal poorly. This is not generally covered by insurance unless there is skin infection or difficulty walking.

For further information, visit the Plastic Surgery Information Service website at **http://www.plasticsurgery.org**. The American Society of Plastic Surgeons and the Plastic Surgery Educational Foundation sponsor this site.

35
To All "Significant Others"

My name is Frank Thompson and I am the husband of Barbara Thompson, the author of this book. I asked Barbara for some space in this book to talk to all the husbands, wives, mothers, fathers, boyfriends, girlfriends or any other "significant other." If a loved one of yours has asked you to read this chapter, congratulations on doing so. I have gone through, and survived, what you are probably experiencing now and I know that I can offer some words that will help you to deal with it.

About two years ago, our family doctor recommended that my wife see a nutritionist about her weight. The nutritionist suggested several plans for her to lose weight, most of which were the standard: more exercise, better eating habits, identifying why people eat emotionally, and taking prescribed weight loss medication. One of the suggestions, however, was for her to have weight loss surgery. I was shocked. How could this man come up with this? Does he really know what he is talking about?

My reactions then, were probably the same as your reactions now. I know what most every one of you was thinking when your loved one told you that he or she was considering weight loss surgery. I can hear your thoughts and your words now as I am writing this.

"You are perfectly healthy!"
"This is a major operation!"
"You could die!!"
"What about the family?"
"What about just one more diet?"
"You are not THAT overweight!"
"How can they say that you are morbidly obese?"
"Why do something that will change your life forever?"

I could go on and on. How do I know what went through your mind? I know because I had the very same thoughts and emotions. I think that anyone who finds out that their loved one is "volunteering" to undergo such a serious operation is naturally concerned about the consequences of such a drastic procedure. I use the word "volunteering" because at that time, I did not fully understand the "need" for the operation. I was worried about how this operation would change her life. I was worried about how she would feel when we would go out to dinner with friends or when she would attend a work related function that was centered around food. I was worried about the fact that some surgeon was going to literally change her insides. Cut some parts here. Reconnect some parts there. This surgeon was actually going to re-route my wife's intestines to places that God never thought about. I was horrified. I was scared. I was speechless. And with all my worry about how this would change my wife's life, I also wondered how this would change my own life and our family. How could I eat in front of her without making her feel bad about not being able to eat more? How could we go out for dinner and a movie? How would I go on if she had complications and died? It is amazing how many thoughts go through your head when you are panicking about the health of your loved one.

> *Cut some parts here. Reconnect some parts there. This surgeon was actually going to re-route my wife's intestines to places that God never thought about.*

After I got over the initial shock, I was able to think a little more rationally and talked over the options with Barbara. After hearing what she had to say, I still could not accept the fact that she needed such a serious procedure. After much discussion, I talked her into trying another diet. I would help. I would go on a diet with her. I would do anything to avoid the operation. Being the wonderful person she is, she agreed to try one more time. She went on another diet and watched what she ate. She went to nutrition classes. She exercised. She did all the things that the nutritionist originally suggested except for the surgery. She did lose some weight but she was not happy and was in constant pain from her back. This is when I started to learn about something called "co-morbidities."º

Many times when people are overweight, there are usually other problems happening now or problems that will develop in the future. Barbara was in a car accident many years ago and has had back pain ever since. The increased weight on her body was not allowing her to live life without pain. Some days the pain was less. Some days the pain was more severe. But there was always pain. This additional problem that is associated with the weight is called co-morbidity. Being overweight makes a person vulnerable to many other problems like diabetes, high blood pressure, heart attacks and something called sleep apnea, when the person actually stops breathing when they sleep. Barbara didn't have any of these other problems then, but being overweight made her a prime candidate for developing these problems in the future.

Another problem that is not normally a co-morbidity is "quality of life." Barbara was not happy about her weight problem and the ever-present back pain. She missed going shopping with our daughter, Erin, because she could only walk for a short time at the malls. She felt bad that she could never fit into the slinky outfits that she wore many years ago. She loves playing golf, but her back would be screaming at her after playing only nine holes. Playing 18 holes of golf was absolutely out of the question. She was taking prescribed and over-the-counter pain medication, going to a chiropractor several times a week, and even got treated several times at a pain center at a local hospital. She was told that the treatments would give her some temporary relief but would not cure her problem, as long as she was heavy.

I looked her in the eyes and I knew in that moment that we were about to take a new direction in our lives.

The turning point for me to accept weight loss surgery was one day when I found Barbara in the kitchen, and in especially great pain. She was crying and sitting in a chair with her head hanging low. She looked up at me with her beautiful blue eyes that were now red and full of tears, and said that she was tired of being in pain all the time and wanted to go ahead with the surgery. My heart melted. I looked her in the eyes and I knew in that moment that we were about to take a new direction in our lives. I could not continue to see the person I love most in this world, in so much pain and I could see that weight loss surgery was the only way to ever find an end to her misery.

Barbara had the pain, but your loved one may only be overweight. My use of the word "only' should not be taken as an indication that there is not a grave problem. To be considered for weight loss surgery, the patent is normally required to be 100 pounds or more over their ideal weight. We have a cat and buy kitty litter in 33 pound containers. To get a full appreciation of what an extra 100 pounds feels like, I suggest that you try strapping three of those containers to your belt. Now spend a couple of hours trying to live your life. I would not be surprised if you gave up after only a few minutes.

As the years go by and the person you love gets heavier and heavier, (which is typically what happens), co-morbidities will surely develop. At some point, you and your loved one will be faced with the horrendous fact that the weight will never come off with conventional means, and the quality of life will deteriorate to the point that there will be a spiral down hill to early death. With every passing day you will notice only small changes and think that there is not a big problem. But things will be slowly getting worse until one day there will be a terrible disaster. It is absolutely critical that something be done to manage the weight problem and it must be done now. Any further delay will only add to your loved one's misery and mounting health problems.

If weight loss surgery has been recommended to your loved one, I urge you from the bottom of my heart, to open your mind to the seriousness of the problem. Make an effort to educate yourself about all aspects of the surgery. Keep in mind that your loved one is in physical and emotional misery and desperately needs your help.

216

Appendix A
Suggested Readings

Atkins, Robert C., Dr. Atkins New Diet Revolution. NY, National Book Network, 1999.

Eades, Michael R., Protein Power: The High Protein/Low Carbohydrate Way to Lose Weight, Feel Fit and Boost Your Health - in Just Weeks! NY, Bantam Books, 1997.

Gawain, Shakti, Creative Visualization. Los Angeles, New World Library, 1995.

Heller, Rachael, Carbohydrate Addict's Carbohydrate Counter. NY, Signet, 2000.

Hansen, Vikki, Seven Secrets of Slim People. NY, Harpercollins, 1999.

Huddleston, Peggy, Prepare for Surgery, Heal Faster: A Guide of Mind-Body Techniques. NY, Christiane Northrup, 1996.

Huddleston, Peggy, Prepare for Surgery, Heal Faster: Relaxation/ Healing Audio Tape. NY, Christiane Northrup, 1998.

Maple, Stephen M., Complete Idiot's Guide to Wills and Estates (Complete Idiot's Guide). NY, MacMillan Distribution, 1997.

Nelson, Miriam E., Strong Women Stay Slim. NY, Bantam Books, 1998.

Netzer, Corinne T., The Complete Book of Food Counts. NY, Dell, 2000.

Orin, Rhonda D., <u>Making Them Pay: How to Get the Most from Health Insurance and Managed Care</u>. NY, St. Martin's Griffin, 2001.

Phillips, Bill, <u>Body for Life: 12 Weeks to Mental and Physical Strength</u>. NY, Harpercollins, 1999.

Steward, H. Leighton, <u>Sugar Busters!: Cut Sugar to Trim Fat</u>. NY, Ballantine Books, 1998.

Warda, Mark, <u>How to Make Your Own Will: With Forms (Self-Help Law Kit with Forms)</u>. N Y, Sourcebook Trade, 1997.

Appendix B
Interesting Web Sites

I have found the following web links to be very helpful to my preparation for surgery and general knowledge about it.

Weight Loss Surgery Center.com
http://www.wlscenter.com
This is my personal website where I have detailed my weight loss surgery journey and included my before and current pictures and statistics. Additionally, you will find weight loss surgery research material and frequently asked questions. My site also recognizes the worldwide community of people who are going through their own weight loss journeys. We celebrate those who have reached the goal of 100 pounds lost. I would appreciate if you would let me know how you liked this book by leaving me a comment in my guest book.

Association for Morbid Obesity Support
http://www.obesityhelp.com/morbidobesity
This site is designed to provide a link to all of the people exploring weight loss surgery. Current membership totals more than 120,000. It is necessary to register on this site in order to explore it, but membership is free. Here you will find local peers along with their experiences, surgeons in your area complete with extensive comments from patients, before and after photos, a clothing exchange, extensive journals of those taking the weight loss surgery journey, and a section devoted to those who have died from surgery.

Obesity Surgery Support Group (OSSG)
http://groups.yahoo.com/group/OSSG
This is an online bulletin board whose purpose is to discuss and offer support for the physical and emotional issues as they relate to weight loss surgery for the morbidly obese. Topics covered include types of surgeries available, dietary guidelines, post-op reports, and

emotional, family, work, and recovery issues. Currently there are over 5,000 members. It is necessary to join this list to access it, but membership is free. This group is the "mother" list, but there are additional OSSG groups that you can also join that have smaller memberships. These include geographically regional groups as well as groups for special subjects such as recipes, living alone, those who are more than one year post-op, and insurance questions. You may "lurk" or post to any of these lists after you have joined. Emails are received singly or in digest form. Previous messages can be accessed from the archives.

American Society for Bariatric Surgery
http://www.asbs.org
This is the professional organization for surgeons performing weight loss surgery. Here you can find surgeons in your area who perform this surgery. This site has extensive research information, especially on types of surgeries available. It also includes a BMI calculator.

The Obesity Law and Advocacy Center
http://www.obesitylaw.com/index.htm
The Obesity Law and Advocacy Center is a full-service private law firm devoted to representing morbidly obese persons in a variety of legal matters. They are especially effective in representing you against your insurance company when you have been denied coverage for your surgery.

UPMC Health System Minimally Invasive Surgery
http://www.upmc.edu/obesitysurgery
This is the site for my surgeon, Dr. Philip Schauer, of Pittsburgh, PA. In the site he discusses obesity and the laparoscopic surgical treatment for morbid obesity

Obesity Online
http://www.obesity-online.com
This is an online magazine that provides current research articles dealing with obesity. Provides very interesting reading.

American Obesity Association
http://www.obesity.org
This is an informative site that discusses obesity and its effects. The Association is devoted to advocacy, research and education.

Beyond Change
http://www.beyondchange-obesity.com
Beyond Change is published monthly by J.K.S. Associates to inform, educate, support and encourage the obese individual, many of whom are in weight management programs or those who have had or perhaps planning to have bariatric (obesity) surgery. The publication offers advice from professionals, information on the most current treatments of obesity, and in general, provides avenues that would allow individuals the ability to make informed choices.

Spotlight Health: Morbid Obesity, Carnie Wilson
http://www.spotlighthealth.com/morbid_obesity/mo/mo.htm
Daughter of legendary Beach Boy Brian Wilson takes us on a journey through her thoughts and feelings as she meets with several specialists, including endocrinologists, surgeons, psychologists, physiatrists and nutritionists on her way to her difficult decision to undergo gastric bypass surgery.

Plastic Surgery Information Service
http://www.plasticsurgery.org/index.cfm
This site is sponsored by the American Society of Plastic Surgeons and the Plastic Surgery Educational Foundation. Here you can find extensive authoritative information about plastic surgery including a search by procedure, a list of plastic surgeons, and average costs per procedure.

Fast Food Facts
http://www.ag.state.mn.us/consumer/health/fff.asp
This is a fast food database with an interactive search form that allows you to find the nutritional values of over 700 menu items from fast food restaurants.

Cyberdiet.com
http://www.cyberdiet.com

Cyberdiet.com is a diet and nutrition website. The site includes nutritional information, interactive tools, and support groups. The self-assessment section includes a nutritional profile. The diet and nutrition section has a daily food planner and a section on dining out. The exercise section allows you to chart your activities.

Appendix C
Appeal Letter

The following is an example of a letter of appeal for insurance coverage. Feel free to use any parts of this letter that may apply to you. All documents and articles cited as exhibits are available either on the internet or from interlibrary loan at your local library. For studies that apply to other co-morbidities, ask your reference librarian to assist you in finding them. You will need to get letters of support and documentation from your own doctors. An appeal package such as this may seem an overwhelming task. But if you are desperate and motivated, you can do it!

To whom it may concern;

I am writing to appeal the denial of my request for coverage of gastric bypass Roux en-Y surgery, Denial # _____, dated _____.

I am a 52 year old female, 5' 6" tall, weighing 365 pounds. Calculating my height in relationship to my weight classifies me as morbidly obese with a Body Mass Index of 59. On page 63 of the XYZ Insurance Company Policy for RTC Corporation there is an exclusion which reads: "Including surgical operations and medical procedures for the treatment of morbid obesity, unless determined to be medically necessary by XYZ Insurance Company." What follows is documentation of why this surgery should be considered a medical necessity for me.

I was first diagnosed with sleep apnea in 1996. I have included a letter of support and medical necessity from my pulmonologist, Dr. Ali as well as results from my polysomnography study conducted December 1995 (see attached Exhibit A). Sleep apnea is a respiratory disease caused when an enlarged abdomen presses against the diaphragm and when the thickened tissues of the neck and chest constrict the airway. Sleep apnea can result in sudden death while sleeping and leads to sleepiness during the day because of constant awakening during the night as the patient gasps for air. Sleepiness can make driving unsafe and hinder work performance. Attached as Exhibit B is an article from the March 2001 issue of the <u>American Journal of Respiratory and Critical Care Medicine</u> which discusses a study associating sleep apnea to obesity. Attached as Exhibit C is the article, "Sleep Disturbance and Obesity," <u>Archives of Internal Medicine</u>, Jan. 8, 2001, p. 102-107, which concludes that sleep apnea is improved with weight loss.

I was also diagnosed with adult onset diabetes in 1998. Included is a report (Exhibit D) from my endocrinologist, Dr. Scott, as well as his letter of support for my surgery. Currently I take 100 units of NPH insulin daily as well as 50 units of Lispro insulin. Diabetes is a fatal disease that takes a terrible toll on the body. In the Sept. 1995 issue of the <u>Annals of Surgery</u>, Dr. W.J. Pories describes the elimination of diabetes in his weight loss surgery patients in the article, "Who Would Have Thought It? An Operation Proves To Be the Most Effective Therapy for Adult-onset Diabetes Mellitus," (Exhibit E). I want a chance to be among those diabetes patients who have the surgery and have a chance for those types of results.

Additional co-morbidities that I have that are caused by or aggravated by my morbid obesity include:
- Pain in my ankles, feet, legs and lower back
- Edema in my ankles, feet and lower legs
- Shortness of breath
- Insomnia
- Migraine headaches
- Urinary incontinence
- Depression

I have been overweight for more than 20 years. During that time, I have tried many diets. I have been a member of Weight Watchers during most of that time and am submitting my Weight Watchers attendance books (Exhibit F). I am also submitting a log of my diet history (Exhibit G). As you can see, I have a pattern of dieting, losing weight, and then regaining the weight plus additional pounds. I am also including a letter (Exhibit H) from my family physician, Dr. Baglia, attesting to the fact that I have followed diet plans that he has supplied to me over the years and that he has prescribed the diet drug Meridia to me in the past. I had the same results with those diets; I initially lost weight, but eventually regained the weight plus additional pounds. It is well established that this pattern of losing and regaining weight is very hard on the body. It is very hard psychologically as well. I have failed at dieting over and over, causing me to have a loss of self-esteem and depression. I have also exercised with these diets. However, my morbid obesity is to a point now that exercising is extremely painful.

My family has a history of morbid obesity. My father weighed 315 pounds when he died at the age of 59 from heart disease. My sister who is 5 years younger than I am is obese and suffers from the beginning stages of many of my same co-morbidities.

The National Institutes of Health in their Mar. 25-27, 1991 Consensus Statement (Exhibit I) describes severe obesity as "a chronic intractable disorder" and that the "surgical procedures in use can induce substantial weight loss, and this, in turn, may ameliorate co-morbid conditions." They further state that "Weight reduction surgery has been reported to improve several co-morbid conditions such as sleep apnea and obesity-associated hypoventilation, glucose intolerance, frank diabetes mellitus, hypertension, and serum lipid abnormalities."

The National Institutes of Health in their Consensus Statement further suggests the following main criteria to be used to determine a patient's eligibility for weight loss surgery:

- A Body Mass Index of 40 or above
  My BMI is 59
- Should have a co-morbidity that will be improved by surgery
  My sleep apnea will be improved by weight loss
  My diabetes will be improved by weight loss
- Should have tried to lose weight by conventional means
  I have supplied ample documented diet history

Weight loss surgery is safe and effective. The American Obesity Association in their paper on obesity surgery (Exhibit J) states that "within 30 days of surgery, 93.4% of patients from a national registry reported no complications from surgery." They further state that "In general, 60% of patients with obesity-related medical conditions are no longer on medication for these conditions three years after surgery." In the article "Obesity Surgery – Another Unmet Need," which appeared in the Sept. 2, 2000 issue of the British Medical Journal, (Exhibit K) weight loss surgery is recognized as a safe and effective surgery and the author questions why it is not performed more often. The author states, "Over the past decade both the National Institutes of Health in the United States and the Scottish Intercollegiate Guideline Network have suggested that surgery is the most effective treatment for selected patients who are morbidly obese. Both organizations have recommended that surgery be carried out more frequently." The article further states that "Most patients who are obese are treated with a combination of advice on diet and lifestyle and in some cases with drugs. However, for patients who have morbid obesity (Body Mass Index > 40), this conservative approach is doomed to failure."

My morbid obesity interferes with my performance of the normal and routine tasks of daily living, such as work, household tasks and recreation. A normal task such as grocery shopping is very difficult for me. My morbid obesity limits my ability to walk, climb stairs and to participate in normal activities that require anything beyond minimal effort. I have a somewhat sedentary job, however getting to and from work is increasingly difficult. It is my desire to be able to live a normal life and perform ordinary activities in my daily and family life.

I have done a tremendous amount of research on weight loss surgery. I have learned a lot about this surgery and what it will do for my life. That is why I know I need the surgery. I understand that there are risks involved with the surgery which include death as is possible from any surgery, wound infection, nutritional deficiencies if a vitamin regime is not followed, hernia, infection from a leak in the digestive system, and bowel obstruction. I recognize these risks and the statistical chance of their occurring. However, I also recognize the fact as stated in the British Medical Journal article that "If left untreated, patients who are morbidly obese have only a 1 in 7 chance of reaching their normal life expectancy."

I hope you will agree that all of the above constitutes medical necessity and that you will approve coverage for my surgery.

Sincerely,

Appendix D
Patient Informed Consent Quiz

The National Institutes of Health has set as one of the guidelines to qualify for weight loss surgery, that patients understand the risks and benefits of the surgery. The following quiz is designed to ensure that you understand all of these possible risks and the very important instructions that you must follow after your surgery to ensure your safety and success. It is recommended that you complete this quiz and discuss your answers with your surgeon or an appropriate member of your surgeon's staff. Use the information found in this book or supplied to you by your surgeon to complete this quiz. Remember that if there are any conflicts between the instructions given to you by your surgeon and what is found in this book, your surgeon's instructions should be followed.

1. Name the type of surgery you will be having and provide a description in your own words of what your surgeon will be doing in the surgery.

2. Name 4 complications that can occur with weight loss surgery.
     1)
     2)
     3)
     4)

3. Is there a risk of death with weight loss surgery? ___Yes ___No.

4. Describe any specific instructions from your surgeon concerning eating and drinking during the first month following surgery.

5. What are some of the danger signs immediately following surgery that you should report immediately to your surgeon?

6. What is the maximum amount of weight that you can lift during the first two weeks following surgery?

7. When can you return to work?

8. What are your specific instructions about taking your regularly prescribed medication just prior to and following your surgery?

9. What are the 4 Rules of Success?
    1)
    2)
    3)
    4)

10. What does "weight loss surgery is only a tool" mean?

11. What is the "Window of Opportunity?"

12. How might your life change following surgery?

13. How often should I visit my surgeon following surgery?

14. What vitamins should I take following surgery?

_____   _____
Patient's Signature   Surgeon's Signature

_____
Date

Bibliography

Alvarado Center for Surgical Weight Control, <u>Surgical Operations for Morbid Obesity</u>. **http://www.gastricbypass.com**, August 21, 2000.

American Society of Bariatric Surgeons, <u>The Story of Surgery for Obesity, Chapter 4, The Mason Era</u>. **http://www.asbs.org**, August 22, 2000.

American Society of Plastic Surgeons and Plastic Surgery Educational Foundation. <u>Treatment of Skin Redundancy Following Massive Weight Loss.</u>
http://www.plasticsyrgery.org/profinfo/pospap/skin.htm, Sept. 2, 2000.

Atkins, Robert C., M.D., <u>Dr. Atkins' New Diet Revolution</u>. New York, Avon Books, 1992.

"Attorney Debates Weighty Issues for Obese Clients," <u>Pittsburgh Tribune Review</u>, Aug. 2, 2000, Style, p. 1.

Balsiger, Bruno, M.D., et al, "Prospective Evaluation of Roux-en-Y Gastric Bypass as Primary Operation for Medically Complicated Obesity." <u>Mayo Clinic Proceedings</u>, Vol. 75, 2000, p. 673-680.

Baxter, John, "Obesity Surgery – Another Unmet Need." <u>British Medical Journal</u>. Vol. 321, Sept. 2, 2000, p. 523-524.

Burge, Jean C., Scahumberg, Joann Zorman, "Changes in Patients' Taste Acuity Roux-en-Y Gastric Bypass for Clinically Severe Obesity," <u>Journal of the American Dietetic Association</u>. Vol. 95, Issue 6, June 1995, p. 666-670

DeMaria, Eric, MD, Sugerman, Harvey, MD, et al. "High Failure Rate After Laparoscopic Adjustable Silicone Gastric Banding for Treatment of Morbid Obesity." Annals of Surgery, Vol. 233, June 2001, p. 808-818.

Dr. Whitaker's Natural Solutions to Osteoporosis, Osteoporosis. http://www.drwhitaker.com/wit_con_osteop.php, August 30, 2000.

Eckel, Robert H., M.D., Obesity and Heart Disease. Dallas, American Heart Association, 1997.

Gallagher, Sharon and R. Armour Forse. "Gastric Bypass", Diabetes Forecast, Vol. 47, Issue 12, Dec. 1994, p. 52-57.

Lew, E.A., and Garfinkel L. "Variations in Mortality by Weight Among 750,000 Men and Women. Journal of Chronic Disease, Vol. 32, 1979, p. 563-576.

Mayo Clinic Family Health Book. New York, William Morrow, 1990.

Pories, W. J., Swanson, M. S., MacDonald, K. G., et al. "Who Would Have Thought It? An Operation Proves To Be the Most Effective Therapy for Adult-onset Diabetes Mellitus." Annals of Surgery, Vol. 222, Sept. 1995, p. 339-50.

Selinkoff, Paul M., M.D. and Pilcher, John, M.D., Surgery for Morbid Obesity. http://www.sabariatric.com/index.htm, August 21, 2000.

Sjostrom, L., Larsson, B. et al. "Swedish Obese Subjects (SOS). Recruitment for an Intervention Study and a Selected Description of the Obese State. International Journal of Obesity Related Disorders, Vol. 16, Issue 6, 1992, p. 465-479.

"Surgery for Severe Obesity," http://www.thriveonline.com/weight/drugs/surgery.html#options, Dec. 5, 1998.

Warkentin, Donald L., M.D., <u>Obesity and the Heart</u>. Clinical Reference Systems, 1998.

"Who Should Consider Gastric Bypass?" <u>Washington Post,</u> Feb. 29, 2000, p. Z12

Index